The LetSleepHappen Insomnia Workbook Series:

Unlearning Insomnia & Sleep Medication Dependence

Rosemary Clancy

The LetSleepHappen Insomnia Workbook Series:

Unlearning Insomnia & Sleep Medication Dependence

Contents

Prologue. How will this book help you? How to use this book.   3

Part 1: UNDERSTANDING INSOMNIA
1. **What happens in insomnia** that keeps our system in threat responding   7
2. **Safeguarding behaviours & Conditioning processes** at the core of insomnia   16
3. **Insomnia & Anxiety: the cycle of anxiety** underlying insomnia learning   26
4. **Our Sleep Processes** that will get sleep back on track   36
5. **Attention processes in Insomnia** that maintain threat monitoring   43

Part 2: UNLEARNING INSOMNIA
6. **Essential Habits & Actions** to get sleep back on track   50
7. **Understanding Sleep Beliefs & Expectations**: that drive insomnia   67
8. **Testing Insomnia Beliefs & Expectations**: barriers to change   74
9. **Insomnia Worry & Rumination**   87
10. **Behaviour Change Experiments** on sleep safeguarding and sleep effort   99
11. **Values review: the "Whys"** to help unlearn Insomnia   104

Part 3: UNLEARNING SLEEP MEDICATION DEPENDENCE
12. **Collaborating with your Prescriber: Reducing Prescription Sleep Medication Safely**   113

Further Reading   125

THE INSOMNIA WORKBOOK:
UNLEARNING INSOMNIA AND SLEEP MEDICATION DEPENDENCE

PROLOGUE:
HOW WILL THIS BOOK HELP YOU?

I am assuming anyone coming to this book has a pretty strong belief they have an insomnia diagnosis. Often they have done a sleep study that confirms it. The people who I see for insomnia Cognitive Behaviour Therapy have generally read a great deal on this problem, which can be both very helpful and not so helpful in starting treatment collaboration. So I deal briefly with insomnia diagnosis, compare it with "normal" sleep (which is a range) and then get on with unfolding the treatment process which guides this workbook layout.

Why does insomnia matter? Because of its prevalence in the community and links with depression and anxiety. Around 30% of the general population reports suffering at least one symptom of insomnia, whether it's trouble falling asleep, staying asleep during the night, or too-early morning waking. Sleep problems and mental health problems are strongly linked. 40-50% of insomnia sufferers have a comorbid mental health disorder. Those with insomnia are ten times more likely to have clinical depression than those without insomnia, and seventeen times more likely to have clinical anxiety. Pre-existing insomnia is a primary risk factor for first episode depression. Sleep loss generates relapse for bipolar I patients, leading to months spent in recovery for many.

In parallel, the number of prescriptions for sleep medications is rising, and along with this the rate of accidental overdose and complex behaviours both risky and unrecalled. A safe and effective longterm treatment for insomnia is sorely needed and universally sought. The effective insomnia treatment involves a combination of acceptance strategies, as well as thinking, attention and behaviour changes.

INSOMNIA FIRST, MEDICATION TAPERING AFTER
About 90% of this book is on learning about and managing sleep disturbance in insomnia. It is 10% about managing and safely reducing sleep medications usage in insomnia. For most people, reducing prescription sleep medications and trusting the brain to regulate sleep probably won't happen until they feel reassured enough they'll get decent sleep without the backup. This is especially if they've been reliant on sleeping pills longterm. So this workbook is largely about learning sleep habits and skills to redevelop trust in the brain's ability to manage sleep on its own.

So this is primarily an insomnia workbook rather than a medication reduction workbook. I am stating this now so you don't feel surprised that the actual nuts and bolts of reducing medications is at the tail-end of the book. This is for a reason: I want to communicate to insomnia sufferers that there is a **process** to work through to build a habit of good sleep. There's no quick fix in insomnia.

The psychological groundwork needs doing before starting to reduce doses in order to 1) give you time to organise your **obligatory** medical supervision beforehand, collaborating on the schedule details with your prescribing practitioner); and 2) give you enough reassurance that you don't panic about sleep loss and vary your dosage wildly. Sudden large drops in dosage tend to be followed by sudden large increases due to panic. Kneejerk self-medicating when panicking about insomnia would probably also scare your prescribing doctor.

The psychological therapy beforehand will mean you will be properly prepared and committed to safely reducing in collaboration with your prescriber. Your expectations will have adapted and your fear levels will be reduced, so you're more likely to keep to the tapering program, and see longterm success. When you're reassured by sound sleep habits forming without having to be forced then your mind can let go of control and let sleep happen in the background.

OVERVALUING SLEEP AND SAFEGUARDING IT

Most people with insomnia who've problem-solved with sleep prescription medication will recognise themselves in the experiences described here. For most people with insomnia sleep medications dependence is not about getting a buzz or euphoria. Sleep medications dependence is about safeguarding sleep. It comes from valuing sleep very highly, even overvaluing sleep, not being reckless with it. This safeguarding of sleep, or sleep "safety-seeking", is a very careful and anxiety-provoking pursuit. As far from euphoria as you could imagine, it's very hard work and day-and-night mental effort and focus.

Valuing sleep is good. Sleep is important for our physical and mental health. We should respect sleep. But overvaluing sleep costs. If we start to fear sleep (when we don't need to) we want to step in and control it manually, instead of letting our brain drive it on autopilot. This effort will routinely fail to make sleep happen, and in fact will make us distrust it more. So this book is about reassuring you with information about your brain's ability to "do" sleep. It features enough information to answer your fears about sleep, and make it easier to let go of your sleep medications in a safe and gradual way. So you can genuinely accept and allow yourself to give over control of your brain's sleep function.

SLEEP DISTURBANCE UNDERPINS MULTIPLE PROBLEMS

This workbook is going to look at sleep disturbance and sleep worries underlying a number of diagnoses. In this way it's "transdiagnostic". People with anxiety disorders have sleep disturbance and daytime tiredness, as do people with major depression, people with mood disorders like Bipolar Affective Disorder, people with chronic worry, with psychotic disorders, with Obstructive Sleep Apnoea. Even people without these disorders have sleep disturbance and daytime tiredness. Because pretty much everyone will have sleep disturbance and worry about sleeplessness at some point.

Even if you've successfully completed a cognitive behavioural insomnia treatment, you will still at times have what you right now call "poor" sleeps. The difference is you'll respond differently to them psychologically compared to before; you'll generally think about them differently. Throughout our lives it's common for humans to experience "good" and "bad" and "mediocre" sleeps. This fact needs acceptance if you're going to be resilient. The possibility of insomnia will always be there, simply because we will still spend around a third of our lives involved in sleep and attending to it, and life stress can't be eradicated completely.

Sleep disturbance is now recognised as a mechanism in causing symptoms and functional disability in multiple psychiatric problems (eg, mood, anxiety, dementia, schizophrenia, eating, chronic pain and substance abuse disorders). Sleep disturbance is closely linked to emotion regulation (Harvey, Murray, Chandler, Soehner, 2010). In all of the above physical and mental health problems, people showed reduced total sleep times, reduced sleep efficiency (percent of time in bed spent asleep), and increased time to fall asleep.

In this way providing information and skills to reshape expectations and form good sleep habits can be a "transdiagnostic treatment", able to reduce sleep disturbance effectively across a range of psychiatric problems. And even indirectly ease symptoms of the associated mood or anxiety problem. Sleep problems and mood problems are what's called "bidirectional". When sleep is disturbed, mood is disturbed. When sleep is improved, mood is improved.

HOW TO USE THIS BOOK
This workbook layout is designed to help you understand and deal with one difficulty at a time, in the following way:
Part 1: UNDERSTANDING INSOMNIA
1. A quick view of **what happens in insomnia** to our thoughts, attention, emotions and actions that keeps our whole system pulled into threat responding
2. The **safeguarding behaviours** at the core of insomnia, when we want to control sleep and don't trust our brains to do it. Understanding the **conditioning processes** underlying our thoughts, feelings and behaviours.
3. The **cycle of anxiety** underlying insomnia learning and conditioning; our brain's oldest balancing act: to 1) help you survive, and 2) get you to sleep.
4. Our **sleep processes - the homeostatic and circadian drives** that look after sleep and will get sleep back on track. We will look at the normal circadian sleep wake cycle and when things go off-track.
5. Understanding how **attention processes & biases** in insomnia maintain threat monitoring, unexpected insights from tinnitus treatment, and how to turn down or reframe noise threats in insomnia.

Part 2: UNLEARNING INSOMNIA
6. The **essential actions and habits you will need to take** to get sleep back on track and let your brain get on with its sleep regulation job.
7. **Understanding sleep beliefs and expectations**: the "shorthand" thinking we do to cope with sleep loss and why it makes sense, but also pulls us into further insomnia, driving sleep-safeguarding actions that backfire.
8. **Testing sleep belief and expectation barriers** to change, and gathering reassuring evidence that can help us uncover biases and unlearn insomnia thinking.
9. **Insomnia Worry & rumination**- the functions of worry, using a worry log, worry session and Rumination management skills to unlearn the bed=worry and rumination association.

10. **Behaviour Change experiments** on sleep safeguarding and sleep effort, to unlearn insomnia habits and thinking.
11. **Values review: the "Whys" that make it possible to do difficult habit changes,** to serve a longer term goal. The choice points that will arise every day to challenge your beliefs and reinforce your values

Part 3: UNLEARNING SLEEP MEDICATION DEPENDENCE

12. **Collaborating with your prescriber to reduce prescription sleep medication safely.** Consulting with your medical practitioner at the start of the process and working through this as a team. Discussions on gradual outpatient tapering or inpatient detox in longterm prescription medication dependence.

CHAPTER 1 UNDERSTANDING INSOMNIA

The experience of medication dependence in insomnia, how it starts up, and how it keeps going. Targeting overthinking and overvaluing sleep, constantly monitoring sleep threats, and "safety-seeking" self-medicating actions that backfire to keep insomnia going.

After a big week packed with work, you've been conscientious and begun your Thursday bedtime routine at 8pm. You've wound down with a warm shower and now settling down with a good book. You filled a prescription for sleep medication 2 months ago and tried to use it only 3 nights a week, because Monday, Tuesday and Thursday are your worst days, and the nights before are your worst sleeps. Your eyelids are getting heavy, everything's moving in the right direction. You miss your place in the book and feel good because you probably don't need to take a sleeping pill. You turn the bedside lamp off and the bedroom is dark. You close your eyes, listening to the muffled sound of traffic in the distance.
Ten minutes later you realise you've been thinking about a meeting tomorrow, and now you feel more awake. You've already taken medication on 3 nights this week and you don't want to take it a fourth night. Especially as last night it didn't work as well as it did Sunday night.
Your mind starts racing with thoughts about how unfair this is, since everything was going according to plan. You've done everything right – the daytime exercise, the wind-down period. Ten minutes ago your eyelids were heavy and sleep was overtaking you. Now your brain is active, rapidly scrolling through next day's work demands and thinking about where you can reschedule meetings and conserve energy if tonight's going to be a bad-sleep night. Your heart rate increases, you start to feel hot and prickly, the feelings of frustration and anxiety escalate.

The next half hour is spent tossing and turning, plumping up the pillows because your neck and is tense and you're worried about getting a headache, calculating how many sick days you've had off work this year, and whether it looks bad to take another one. You get up to go to the toilet because your bladder is one thing you can manage to eliminate sleep threats. At the end of the half hour, even though you've resisted it, you take a Valium. It seems to work less well than yesterday evening. You feel some relief after you've taken it because it has worked so far to get you off to sleep, and now you're not trying to do it on your own. But a part of your brain is also assessing whether it's working as well now, after 4 days of using it this week.

During the rest of the night you get a block of sleep then what seems to be semi-conscious drifting. When the alarm goes off you wake groggy, headachey, woolly-headed and still a bit sedated. You feel depleted and fatigued yet strangely anxious and desperate, fearing that there's no guarantee the next night's sleep will be any better. A hot shower and strong coffee do help to freshen you up, but during the day you make some minor mistakes and each time your focus goes straight to last night's sleep as the reason.

By 3pm you want a coffee because of the exhaustion, but immediately think about its effects on tonight's sleep. Your shoulders and neck are wound-up tight and you want to get out and run but too-late exercise affects sleep as well, so no exercise after 4pm. The trapped feeling adds to the tired and wired state. For someone who was always organized, good at taking control and problem-solving you sure feel powerless right now. How can sleep go so wrong when you're trying so hard to do everything right?

This night and day preoccupation with poor sleep and tiredness, and trying to resolve it, sets up a frustrating struggle that is the core of insomnia: the harder you try to make sleep work, the worse it gets.

This workbook directly targets this paradox of insomnia: how desperate efforts to "make" sleep happen (with medications or any other sleep aids) actually create a hyperfocus on your sleep and worsen it. But with a few good tools you'll be able to release yourself from this struggle, and get better sleep without having to rely on sleep medications.

The way out of insomnia involves training core sleep-wake behaviours and thinking that mark good sleep, and starting to understand and work with your brain and body's innate sleep regulation and defence mechanisms. To start off this training let's look at what's needed for an "insomnia" diagnosis.

DO I HAVE INSOMNIA? INSOMNIA CHECKLIST (THE DSM-V DIAGNOSTIC CRITERIA)
In plain English the criteria for assessing insomnia according to the American Psychiatric Association's widely used diagnostic manual (DSM-5th edition) are (please tick off symptoms if you recognize them):

Check	Insomnia symptoms:
✔	Clear dissatisfaction with sleep quantity or quality
	Difficulty initiating, and/or maintaining sleep (frequent waking, or problems resuming sleep after waking); or
	Early morning waking with inability to resume sleep
	Significant distress, impaired social/occupational/ educational / behavioural/ functioning
	At least 3 nights per week, and present for at least 3 months (chronic)
	Occurs despite adequate opportunity for sleep (plenty of time in bed)
	"tired & wired" during the day - daytime fatigue but also tense & edgy
	Daytime poor concentration, thinking & memory impairment
	Insomnia symptoms are not due to the physical effects of a substance
	Insomnia is not better explained by/ does not occur exclusively during, the course of another sleep-wake disorder (eg narcolepsy, Obstructive Sleep Apnoea, Circadian sleep wake disorder)
	Co-existing mental disorders & medical conditions don't adequately explain the main insomnia complaint

Insomnia can be Acute, lasting a few days (Transient insomnia) to 3-4 weeks (short term insomnia; or it can be Chronic: Lasting for more than 1–3 months.

Transient insomnia can be triggered by multiple factors, including:
•Changes to your sleep environment due to physical stimuli (noise, light, movements), or moving to an unfamiliar environment;
•A high state of central nervous system fight-flight activation, triggered by emotional events such as ongoing worry, anxiety, pain, illness, grief, and even excitement;
•inadequate sleep hygiene: including irregular sleep-wake patterns, and continued side effects of stimulants that delay sleep; and/or
•Short-term disruption of your circadian rhythm or body clock brought on by rotating shift work or jetlag.

It's important to check the problem you're seeking help for is insomnia and not another type of sleep disorder.

OTHER SLEEP DISORDERS

Some people may have what appears to be insomnia but there's also something else complicating the picture, like sleepwalking or excessive daytime sleepiness, or nightmares, or flashbacks to previous trauma. Keeping a sleep diary, like the one following, is a good way to gather information. If you note down any unusual symptoms then make an appointment to talk with your doctor about them.

It could be a breathing-related sleep problem with snoring, gasping, airway difficulties, and daytime sleepiness. Or perhaps Periodic Limb Movements, parasomnias (which include sleepwalking, sleeptalking, confusion and night terrors); teeth grinding and associated jaw pain and temporo-mandibular headaches; or nightmares. There could be unusual symptoms representing Narcolepsy (sudden sleep attacks without warning, collapsing or extreme muscle weakness triggered by emotion, a picture of breakthrough REM sleep into waking); or hallucinations or strange sensations when fall asleep or waking. Or even temporary paralysis upon waking.

There are evidence-based behaviour treatments to help other sleep disorders, but you would need to clarify diagnostically with a sleep/respiratory physician what's going on for you medically first (usually via a sleep study). For Sleep-related breathing disorders a behavioural intervention could help you with CPAP device desensitization and for accompanying insomnia; or chronotherapy, timed light and melatonin administration for circadian rhythm sleep-wake disorders; or napping & avoiding sleep deprivation if parasomnias or hypersomnias; or medication timing for Restless Legs Syndrome. Colin Espie's excellent "Overcoming Insomnia and Sleep Problems" book is a great read if you want more detail on these.

KEY ISSUES IN INSOMNIA

The key insomnia issues are difficulty getting to or staying asleep, and daytime tiredness and social and occupational impairment. Despite adequate opportunity to sleep (ie enough time spent in bed), and chronically. Most insomnia sufferers feel sleep deprived but are not sleepy during the day; they're more "tired and wired". It's important that you assess the type and severity of your sleep problem to get the right help, rather than just chronically suffering in silence (given the sheer volume of our lives devoted to sleep), and because some of the sleep disorders can have serious health risks if left untreated.

WHAT'S THE DIFFERENCE BETWEEN MY SLEEP NOW AND THE SLEEP I WANT?

How do we know if a treatment has worked and we have good quality sleep? And how to measure it? As Colin Espie states: through self-report, behavior and physiological data-gathering.

Self-report: Colin Espie describes how Sleep "Quality" by definition needs to be assessed with self-reporting (eg Sleep Questionnaires and sleep diaries) as it measures subjective assessment by us individuals about whether our sleep is poor or good. According to Nava Zisapel at Tel Aviv University our *subjective perception* of sleep (not just objective sleep quality) has health outcomes. Charles Morin devised the Insomnia Severity Index, and Daniel Buysse devised the Pittsburgh Sleep Quality Index (PSQI- assessing sleep dimensions of Regularity, Satisfaction, Alertness, Timing, Efficiency, and Duration) both of which can be found online to fill in and take along to your doctor.

Behaviour: is measured by Actigraphy (movement-based measurement worn like a wristwatch, where data is stored and later analysed for sleep and wake cycle issues.

Physiological measures: these are measured via polysomnography, comprising electrical activity in the brain or EEG (electroencephalography), muscle activity with EMG (electromyography), and eye movements via electro-oculography (EOG).
The most detailed investigation is done when you stay overnight at a sleep laboratory, or less detailed with a home-based study (you are instructed on how to fit the technology at a sleep clinic and then take the portable apparatus home). The benefit is you may get a truer reading of your sleep habits in your own familiar home environment.

Sleep diary: the act of completing a sleep diary not only promises better understanding of your sleeping patterns, but in itself motivates change in behaviours leading to better sleep, in the same way that completing a food diary motivates change in eating habits. It yields much (often reassuring) information – things that confirm your expectations and things that are unexpected. This is useful for generating an individual sleep plan targeting your insomnia causes. You won't have to do it forever – in the long term we'd like you to ignore your sleep like good sleepers do – but just long enough to learn new skills and see them working.

A sleep diary includes information about how long you think it takes you to get to sleep onset after getting into bed and turning off the lights, any waking after sleep onset during the night (WASOs), quality ratings, and any events or substances that might affect your quality rating.

You just colour in the boxes in first 10 minutes after waking in the morning. You don't have to clock-watch to do this because it's based on your "felt sense" of how many hours were slept. No exactitude is needed, because your consistent perceptions show a pattern emerging over several weeks anyway. Try recording a 2-week baseline on the example diary on the next page:

LetSleepHappen

2 week sleep diary

Please rate your:
Sleep quality /100
Daytime alertness /100
Daytime functioning /100

Please complete the boxes as described here:		exercise		E	medication		M	alcohol		A(2)	Please record number of standard drinks
Waking in the morning	W	Going to bed at night	I	Nap			MM	Food/ snacks	F		
Rising from bed in a.m.	R	Sleeping in bed (home)		Sleeping in bed (away)				Caffeine (coffee/ Cola/etc)	C		
Work hours	—	Toilet visits	T	Unintentional daytime sleep		X					

Week 1

Week 2

Day of the week	Fr												
date													
midday	F												
1300	—												
1400	—												
1500	MM C												
1600													
1700													
1800													
1900	A2												
2000	F												
2100	T												
2200													
2300													
midnight													
0100													
0200	T												
0300													
0400													
0500													
0600	W												
0700	R T M C												
0800	E												
0900													
1000													
1100am													
Rate sleep quality /100													
Rate daytime alertness /100													
Rate daytime functioning /100													

In the meantime, let's look at how insomnia starts up and locks in.

HOW INSOMNIA STARTS AND KEEPS GOING
HOW DOES INSOMNIA START UP? The role of attention and doing stuff to force sleep.
For so many with insomnia the starting point was a few sleepless nights during a period of stress (illness, new job, new baby, shift work) which then resolved, but the sleep loss continued on, drawing in more focused attention, mental problem-solving and emotional stress, until you're on physical and sensory high alert, becoming conditioned in a process Prof Adrian Wells at Oxford says looks like this:

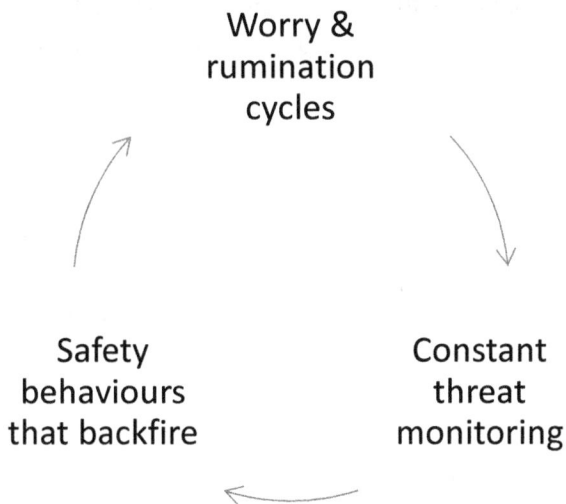

Worry &
rumination
cycles

Safety   Constant
behaviours   threat
that backfire   monitoring

Insomnia maintenance features: worrying and ruminating about sleep loss (*why can't I sleep? how will I function tomorrow? I shouldn't have worked back late!!*) leads to more attention on poor sleep signs (*nighttime wakefulness and alertness*) which leads to problem solving with sleep safeguarding or "safety-seeking" behaviours (*medication, other substances, and other things you do or take, to try to bring on sleep*) which **backfire** by increasing more attention on the problem, more worry about sleep, and so on, in a vicious cycle.

THE 24-HOUR INSOMNIA NIGHTMARE
So the above worry is the night time cycle of insomnia. Unfortunately, you are already aware that insomnia is a 24-hour nightmare. The daytime cycle looks like this: worrying and ruminating (about both poor sleep the night before and daytime tiredness, lack of energy, poor daytime functioning, poor concentration), leads to more attention to all of the above symptoms, leads to safety-seeking actions of cancelling appointments, conserving energy or trying to create energy with stimulants like caffeine.

WHAT KEEPS INSOMNIA GOING
The above cycle becomes conditioned to continue and neural pathways develop to strengthen and expedite the process. Insomnia keeps happening after the original stress resolves with the conditioned process of:

Safety –seeking behaviours:
Night-time safety-seeking behaviours: anything you do during the night to try to bring about sleep, from warm milk to alcohol, toilet visits, nasal sprays, changing sleeping positions repeatedly, herbal teas, taking sleeping medications, even squeezing your eyes tightly closed in a bid to "make" sleep happen. Each one of them is a "sleep experiment" your brain hypothesizes will get you closer to sleep, so it now has to stay alert and monitor if your efforts are working or not. This is called "sleep effort" which makes insomnia worse.

Daytime safety-seeking behaviours are anything you do in the daytime to:
a) conserve energy, like avoiding activities or cancelling appointments, or b) create energy with stimulants like coffee, sugars, cigarettes or stimulant medications. The stimulant effects can last much longer than expected (12 hours after a coffee the stimulant caffeine still affects brain activity), then making it harder to get to sleep. If anxiety about sleep is added to this, the stage is set for more insomnia.

Constant threat monitoring – even before you try a safety-seeking /problem solving behavior, you're already focused on what's going wrong with your sleep (let me count the ways!...) but after you've tried a solution you then have to keep your attention on whether it's working, or well enough. This keeps your attention firing and keeps the problem of insomnia on the front burner. "Good" sleepers don't have their attention on things that are wrong with sleep so they aren't reinforcing a generalized distrust in their brain's ability to regulate sleep.

Worry and rumination processes, where all your analytical skill comes into play, and the good problem-solvers can worry away at this for hours, perking up the frontal lobe (investigating! planning! Strategizing! Executing plans and reviewing!) and preventing the next 70-90 minute sleep cycle from overtaking them. Inevitably insomnia is set to worsen as you try to think ahead of sleep and take control of it. Good sleepers don't even think about this, but if asked they'd probably agree that they leave it to their brain to regulate sleep, at least. That means no need to outthink it, monitor it or "help it along" with any particular aids.

This is not something to beat yourself up about; your best efforts at problem solving have good sleep science behind them (like warm baths, dark rooms, and no electronic devices), and you should validate all this trying, as you learn a lot about sleep in the process.
It's just that insomnia isn't something that can be "solved" in a straightforward way, as the problem solving just becomes part of the generalized "trying too hard". It then creates more hypervigilance, more nervous system activation, more mental alertness.

If you can remember what good sleep felt like you can get back to it, and it won't take long once you start the change and acceptance strategies in this program.   The goal is to overcome the insomnia struggle by valuing sleep but not overvaluing it, not drowning in the desperate sleep effort and attention that adds more threat; just feeling comfort and relief when you get into bed.

Using strategies drawn from evidence-based Cognitive Behaviour Therapy, Mindfulness, and Acceptance & Commitment Therapy principles, this program can bring you measurable, substantial improvement in your sleep and daytime energy and activity levels, targeting:

- **Insomnia:** difficulties in getting to sleep, staying asleep, and/or waking too early in the morning, with poor sleep quality, daytime tiredness, fatigue, irritability, impaired memory and concentration
- **sleep-wake cycles** that are too delayed, too advanced or non-24 hr (eg shift work), with powerful yet inexpensive treatment based on light and dark exposure at different times of the day and night.
- **reducing or ceasing sleep medication**

Briefly, the strategies that work in Cognitive Behaviour Therapy (CBT) are these:

CBT involves **cognitive therapy**, or strategies targeting faulty beliefs, worries, and expectations about sleep and daytime functioning that worsen insomnia; and **behaviour therapy**, or behaviour change strategies that target the unhelpful insomnia habits that you've unintentionally become conditioned to:

The best-practice insomnia and sleep-wake disruption CBT strategies include:

Stimulus control therapy: behaviour change to reassociate the bed environment with sleep and to re-establish a consistent sleep-wake cycle: 1) go to bed when sleepy, 2) get out of bed after 20 minutes when unable to sleep, 3) use the bed only for sleep (no TV, electronic devices), 4) get out of bed at the same time every morning, and 5) don't nap during the day (to build greater pressure to sleep over the day).

Sleep consolidation (time-in-bed restriction) therapy: curtailing time in bed to the actual hours of sleep, to increase sleep efficiency (ie getting the most sleep out of your time in bed). This also ensures you associate your bed environment with sleep instead of waking, and ultimately reducing threat and anxiety about sleep loss.

Relaxation training: exercises to reduce muscle tension, central nervous system activation and racing thoughts which can get in the way of sleep.

Sleep hygiene education: guidelines about lifestyle change (eg diet, exercise, alcohol/substance use) and bed environment change (light, noise, temperature) that can help improve sleep. Also information about what's normal in sleep, and how sleep changes with age.

Sleep diary: completing a sleep diary yields better understanding of your sleeping patterns, and motivates habit change bringing better sleep, providing reassuring information that helps change expectations of sleep "brokenness".

CHAPTER 2   SLEEP SAFEGUARDING BEHAVIOURS THAT BACKFIRE
The insomnia cycle: breaking it down. The sleep hypervigilance loop. How safety-seeking habits form and become automatic. Automatic, conditioned habits you can't think your way out of.

THE INSOMNIA CYCLE: BREAKING IT DOWN
When we are sleepless THOUGHTS lead to FEELINGS lead to ATTENTION lead to ACTIONS, in a sleep "hypervigilance" (hyperalertness) loop:

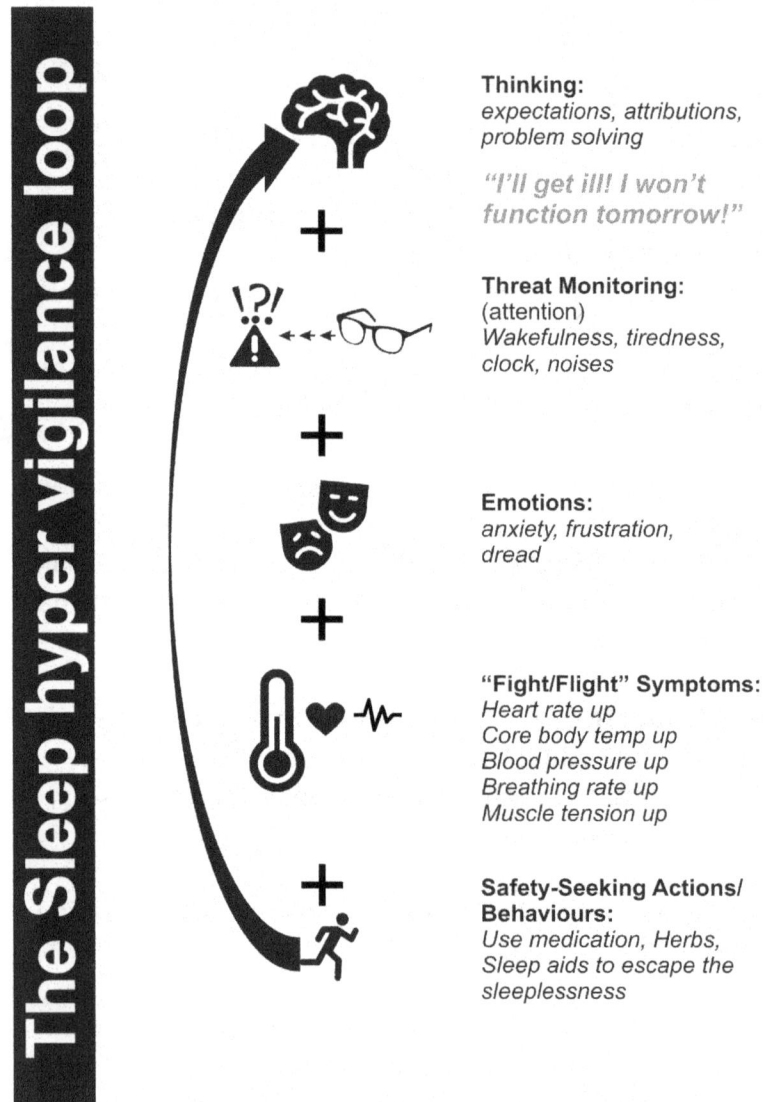

The Sleep hyper vigilance loop

Thinking:
expectations, attributions, problem solving

"I'll get ill! I won't function tomorrow!"

Threat Monitoring:
(attention)
Wakefulness, tiredness, clock, noises

Emotions:
anxiety, frustration, dread

"Fight/Flight" Symptoms:
Heart rate up
Core body temp up
Blood pressure up
Breathing rate up
Muscle tension up

Safety-Seeking Actions/ Behaviours:
Use medication, Herbs, Sleep aids to escape the sleeplessness

THE NIGHT-TIME INSOMNIA CYCLE

Trigger situation: awake in bed at 2am
Leads to:
Threat thoughts "I won't get enough sleep! I won't function tomorrow! I will get sick! I have no control over my sleep!
Leads to:
Emotion: creates 90% Anxiety intensity (a subjective rating of emotion helps you measure change over time), also intense dread and frustration
With the intense anxiety comes intense nervous system "fight-flight" activation to ready you for fleeing or fighting, with physical sensations of anxiety or even panic
Leads to:
Monitoring or scanning for threats in yourself or your environment (wakefulness, tiredness, pain, discomfort, noises)
Leads to:
Attempts to problem-solve with sleep "safety-seeking" behaviours or sleep safeguarding actions, which promise relief from anxiety and sleeplessness and tend to confirm the threat thinking (plus the need to escape distress)
Leads to:
hypervigilance about tiredness and wakefulness that confirms the threatening thoughts.

Reinforcing that it's a 24-hour problem, the daytime cycle of insomnia anxiety looks like this:

THE DAYTIME INSOMNIA CYCLE

Trigger situation: 10am, exhausted at work desk
Leads to:
Worrying thoughts: "I haven't had enough sleep, I feel awful"
"I'm so tired, I don't have the energy to do anything" I wont be able to function today because of last night's sleep" "I'll probably get sacked"
Leads to:
Emotions: anxiety, dread, despair, frustration 90%
Leads to:
Monitoring: of tiredness symptoms, grogginess, aches, error rate, energy level, memory lapses, functioning level
Leads to:
Safety-seeking behaviours/actions: (to safeguard energy)
Stimulants to increase alertness & create energy (caffeine, nicotine, prescription stimulants)
Cancel appointments or ring in sick at work to conserve energy & regain sleep
Naps and reduce commitments to conserve energy
Leads to:
hypervigilance about tiredness and nonalertness that confirms the threatening thoughts.

WHAT DOES <u>YOUR</u> NIGHT-TIME INSOMNIA CYCLE LOOK LIKE?

Night time hyper vigilance loop

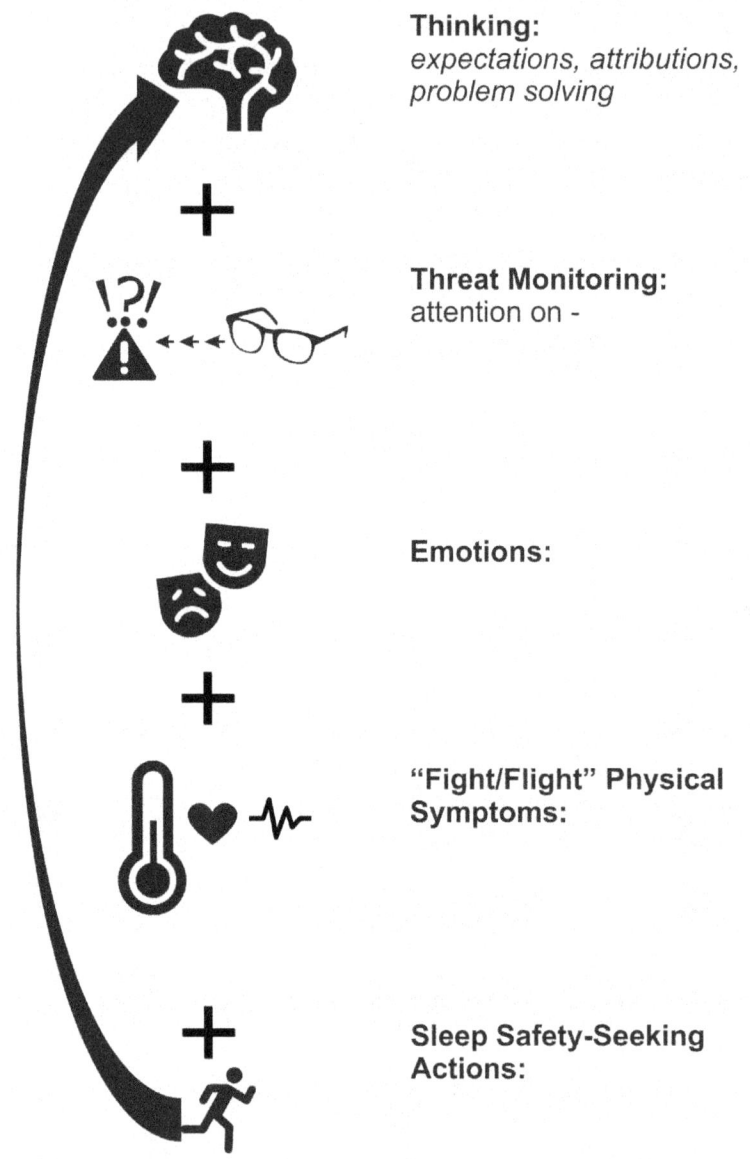

Thinking:
expectations, attributions, problem solving

+

Threat Monitoring:
attention on -

+

Emotions:

+

"Fight/Flight" Physical Symptoms:

+

Sleep Safety-Seeking Actions:

AND WHAT DOES <u>YOUR</u> DAYTIME INSOMNIA CYCLE LOOK LIKE?

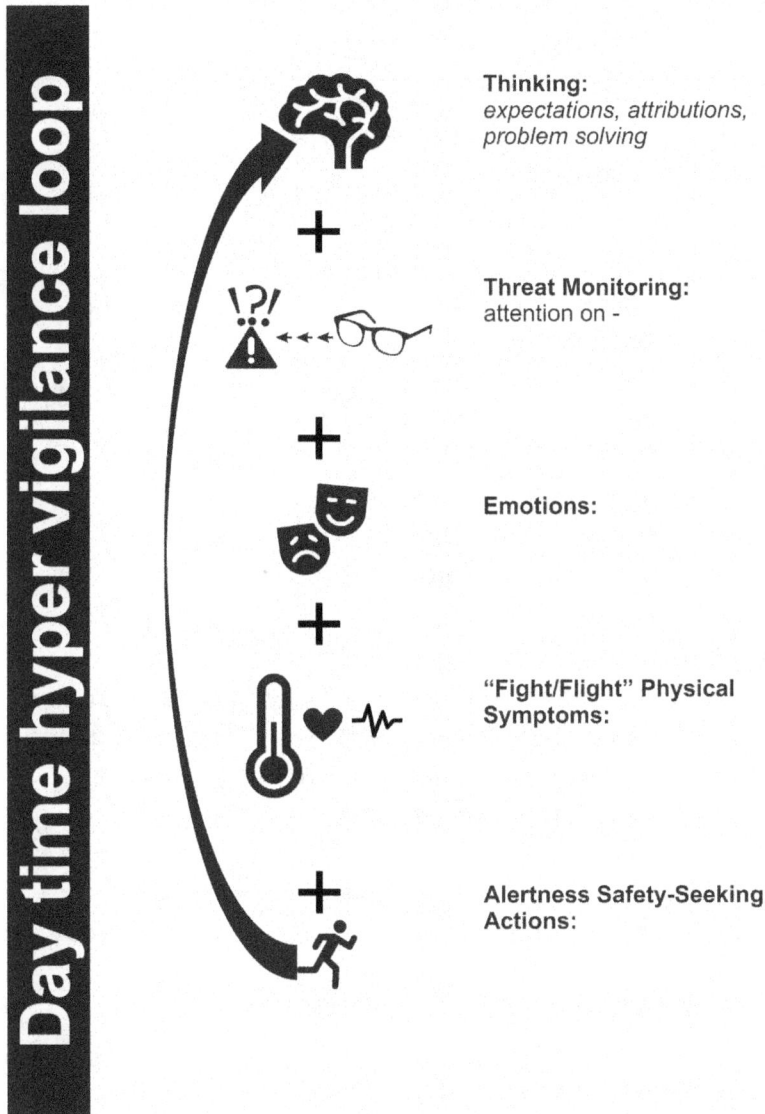

Day time hyper vigilance loop

Thinking:
expectations, attributions, problem solving

+

Threat Monitoring:
attention on -

+

Emotions:

+

"Fight/Flight" Physical Symptoms:

+

Alertness Safety-Seeking Actions:

SAFETY-SEEKING ACTIONS/BEHAVIOURS BACKFIRE TO CREATE MORE THREAT

So the focus needs to be on the night-time sleep safeguarding actions and the daytime alertness/energy safeguarding actions that accidentally create more threat and distrust in our sleep. We're not going to get confidence back in our sleep ability if we've got locked into an automatic habit of hypervigilance, sleep effort, and endless problem-solving with sleep aids.

Let's look at the vast range of safety-seeking actions we do then understand how our brain naturally forms habits that become automatic over time and very hard to get out of.

MY NIGHT-TIME SLEEP SAFEGUARDING/SAFETY-SEEKING ACTIONS CHECKLIST:

	Avoid socialising at night
	Go to bed same time every night without fail
	Go to toilet multiple times before bed & during night
	Avoid drinking water several hours before bed
	Use herbal teas, magnesium, sedatives
	Use alcohol to get to sleep
	Overly-involved bedtime routine with baths, meditation, reading, focused on calming self perfectly but signalling lack of confidence in sleep (eg 45 mins+ bedtime routine)
	Use nasal decongestant sprays so blocked nose won't affect sleep
	Weighted blanket, pillow menu (eg coolgel pillows) to maximise sleep chances, lavender sprays/sachets
	Try to blank out or suppress thoughts when awake in bed
	roll over/ change position/ puff up pillow or turn pillow around in attempt to get back to sleep
	Stay in bed if sleepless, and stay in bed in morning to catch up sleep, keeping room dark
	Over 30 min nap during day (to get more sleep quantity)

You'll notice many of these actually do help sleep, and in many cases (not alcohol or nicotine) have good scientific evidence behind them. These can help if you're using one or two. But if you're ticking off over 70% of the list then you're signalling a lack of confidence in your brain's own sleep processes, and the sheer sleep effort is more likely to increase your performance anxiety and hypervigilance about sleep loss.

And because insomnia is a 24-hour problem, let's look at the range of daytime safety-seeking actions we do to try to safeguard and create alertness and energy during the day.

DAYTIME ENERGY/ALERTNESS SAFEGUARDING ACTIONS CHECKLIST:

	Avoid socialising during the day to conserve energy
	Sit at home on days off watching TV to conserve energy
	Cancel appointments or ring in sick at work to conserve energy & regain sleep
	Use stimulants to increase alertness & energy (caffeine, nicotine, prescription or herbal stimulants)if having to work/ study/socialise, but no coffee or other stimulants after midday to protect sleep
	Have daytime naps + reduce commitments to conserve energy

You can see the daytime actions accidentally create hypervigilance about tiredness and nonalertness that confirms the threatening thoughts of not coping, and the desire to conserve energy at all cost.

The issue with sleep and alertness "safety-seeking" or safeguarding actions is how actions meant to temporarily assist sleep become automatic and habitual.

Charles Duhigg writes on how habits form: every habit starts with a psychological pattern called a "habit loop," a three-part process that has 1) a cue or trigger, that signals your brain to go into automatic mode and let an action or behaviour unfold. Then 2) the routine, the behaviour itself, that we think of as the "habit", and 3) the reward, or something that your brain likes or thinks is important that helps it recall the "habit loop" in the future. Habits are evidence of how efficient our brains are; the brain's way to take a rest, saving us from needing to make endless decisions about the smallest things. 40% of the actions we do daily are the product of habits rather than decisions. But this also means bad habits are difficult to extinguish, as you can see next.

Where this hurts us in insomnia is when our cue of sleeplessness is followed by a behaviour routine that gives us the reward of sleep, so that we get hooked on the safety-seeking habit very quickly.

One example is alcohol to get to sleep. Feared or actual sleeplessness (cue) triggers alcohol intake (behaviour habit) to sedate the nervous system and bring on sleep (reward).

Another example is multiple toilet trips before bed to prevent sleep disruption. Feared sleeplessness (cue) triggers several toilet trips to empty the bladder completely before bed (behaviour habit), anxiety reduces and sleep results (reward).

Another example is nasal decongestant spray use in insomnia. A blocked nose becomes associated with sleeplessness (cue), a decongestant nasal spray is used (behaviour habit) that temporarily shrinks blood vessels inside the nose so it feels like breathing is easier so the nervous system is calmer, and sleep results (reward). So as the habits form there are 2 types of associative learning happening here: operant conditioning and classical conditioning.

Please bear with me while I describe how we learn through these two types of conditioning:
1. **Operant conditioning:** a form of learning where our behaviour is shaped by things that come before (antecedents) and things that come after our behaviour (consequences). Rewards and punishments change the behaviour that follows (first described by B.F. Skinner). So the reward in insomnia safety-seeking habits is anxiety removal and sleep.

    POSITIVE REINFORCEMENT
    This "positive reinforcement" of sleep and calm makes us more likely to repeat the behaviour that produced it, whether it be drinking alcohol, doing multiple toilet trips, using nasal sprays or sleep medications. And when one of those fails to work consistently (called "intermittent reinforcement") our behaviour will *escalate* as we frantically try to make the reward come. Until the reward no longer comes at all, and our behaviour habit faces "extinction".

Also consider what happens when we layer many sleep aids and can't work out with certainty which one actually got us to sleep successfully. Was it a bit of this and maybe a bit of that that worked? Because of the insomnia the sleep reward still seems inconsistent – two nights later the sleep is poor on *all* the sleep aids. This explains why people find it hard to drop *any* of the sleep aids they've layered up "just in case" each resulted in sleep at some point and could work again.

2. **Classical conditioning:** describes the way in which we humans learn by association. Previously neutral signals or stimuli become associated with naturally occurring responses. Anxiety development originates from a learned association between an intrinsically not-aversive event and an expected disaster. An example of this happens at my local Coogee Diggers swimming pool every Saturday. The pool manager puts on Metallica's "Nothing Else Matters" as the last song before the pool closes, and has done for a while now. So I now have a learned association between the previously not-threatening Metallica song and my anxiety about getting my swim in and getting out of the changerooms before closing time.

In insomnia, previously neutral stimuli like the clock and the bed become associated with feared sleeplessness and this unthreatening object then triggers anxiety. In insomnia another neutral stimulus is time: certain hours in the middle of the night where the bed becomes associated with threatening waking and anxiety.

(This came from Ivan Pavlov's experiments in classical conditioning, where he demonstrated how a completely unrelated stimulus can create a response in an organism: a dog would previously salivate at the sight of food, but not at hearing a bell. Pavlov showed how bell-hearing could become a conditioned stimulus paired with the conditioned response of salivating).

What "rewards" or positive reinforcement do I get from my sleep safeguarding actions:
Anxiety or sleep related:
What negatives come from my sleep safeguarding actions:
Anxiety or sleep related:

ASSOCIATIVE LEARNING AND OUR BRAIN'S HABIT-FORMING EFFICIENCY

Neuroscientist Professor David Linden describes the evolutionary adaptive response of our thinking and sensory systems priority of detecting change, and no longer detecting what's static or unchanging. As a result, we will notice something that's novel or unfamiliar to us, but as it becomes familiar to us we acclimatise to its presence and then proceed to ignore it. This is part of our brain's great efficiency and economy. Associative learning reflects this efficiency.

Neuroplasticity writer and researcher Norman Doidge, in The Brain that Changes Itself, talks of this also when he describes that much cortex and focused attention are the starting condition for new learning (such as the great concentration we devote when learning to drive a car) and change in the brain's plasticity. As we repeat a new behaviour we "fire and wire" new neural pathways that make the behaviour habitual and more automatic, using less cortex and less concentration over time. This reflects the incredible efficiency and economy of the brain but also the automaticity that makes it hard to get out of entrenched, conditioned habits.

Charles Duhigg writes in some detail on the decision-making part of our brains working less and less as a behaviour becomes more automatic. As the learned behaviour has become more automatic there is less and less brain capacity burning energy trying to make decisions. This holds for every habit from learning to drive to brushing our teeth before bed. What's great about this automaticity process is your brain is freed up to do complex decision-making in your prefrontal cortex as the brain's basal ganglia takes over the automatic routine.

Duhigg describes how neuroscientists have traced our habit-making behaviours to the basal ganglia, which also plays a key role in the development of emotions, memories and pattern recognition. Decisions, meanwhile, are made in a different part of the brain called the prefrontal cortex. *But as soon as a behaviour becomes automatic habit, the decision-making centre of our brain goes into "sleep mode".*

"In fact, the brain starts working less and less," says Duhigg. "The brain can almost completely shut down. ...it means you have all of this mental activity you can devote to something else." That's why it's easy — eg while driving or parallel parking, which is pretty complex and difficult when you're a learner driver — to completely focus on something else: like singing a song on the radio, or having a conversation with your passenger.

Duhigg explains we can do these complex behaviours without being in the least mentally aware of it. And all because of the ability of our basal ganglia to take a behaviour and turn it into an automatic routine. Once paired associations are familiar and habitual to us, the basal ganglia governs a habit's operation, freeing active decision-making up in frontal lobe.

So now consider this in the automatic sleep safeguarding habits we do, from going to the toilet 4 times before bed, taking a medication, using decongestant nasal sprays, or brushing our teeth as part of the bedtime ritual. We no longer have to think about the actions or make decisions, the habit has quickly become automatic care of our basal ganglia. Now our prefrontal cortex is freed up to problem-solve complex work issues. That's why we're so bewildered when we do all the right sleep-inducing things to bring about sleep, but we've already firmly associated our bed with wakefulness and frustration, which is habitual and doesn't need complex thought. It just happens because it's conditioned to happen. At 11pm bedtime or 2am waking. The only way out is to *action* your way out of a conditioned association, not *think* your way out of it.

MEDICATION ISSUE

The safety action of taking a sleep medication has all the ingredients of habit formation: the cue (sleeplessness), an easy behaviour/action (take a pill) and a reward (nervous system calmative, allowing sleep). It doesn't extinguish easily because even if tolerance is reached and at increasing doses the medication isn't so effective anymore (due to neuroadaptation in the reward pathway) every few days the insomnia sufferer will still get sleep purely because of homeostatic pressure to sleep. This "intermittent reinforcement" (of uncertain on-off sleep "reward") can escalate the habitual dosing behaviour, as the insomnia sufferer takes a second or third desperate medication dose (or worse, adds in alcohol) on poor sleep nights to bring on the reward of anxiety-removal and sleep.

The good news in this is that even if tolerance to the medication has developed, your homeostatic and circadian drives are still faithfully operating in the background like they have for 30,000+ years, despite any distrust you may have about them! After 2 nights of poor sleep your brain can be trusted to assess you're in sleep deprivation and make you sleep despite your need to stay hypervigilant for threat.

Many people think that starting a sleep medication will "break the circuit" of insomnia, after which they will naturally go back to decent sleep. However, they're not *breaking a circuit* by starting the medication, they're *forming a new medication habit* - and grafting it onto the insomnia habit - with a perceived reward of sedation and perceived sleep. This habit is helped by sleep medication's amnesia effect: reduced or no recall of night-time waking. You can understand why attribution change happens so quickly (attributing sleep success to the medication instead of one's own brain, after suffering a period of insomnia).

THE REWARD/POSITIVE REINFORCEMENT OF MEMORY LOSS

So there is a function where benzodiazepine sleep medication offers continuous positive reinforcement (which keeps both the behaviour habit and the attributions of medication necessity going). That helpful function is memory loss. Because even though the medications lose effectiveness over time as sleep-inducers and anti-anxiety agents, according to researchers Vinkers & Olivier they don't lose effectiveness in creating anterograde amnesia (preventing laying down of new memory). (This reinforces a finding raised earlier by Mejo and other researchers).

Lack of tolerance developing to effects of memory loss means we may continue to benefit from forgetting any wakefulness periods during the night. This of course isn't guaranteed, as noted earlier, if you're agitated enough you can be pacing all night and certainly recall that happening: to get to sleep you still need to "collaborate" with the medication (as Glovinsky & Spielman phrase it). But several researchers have noted the different tolerances (and reduced therapeutic effects) that emerge with long term use of benzodiazepines.

THE REINFORCING REWARD SYSTEM
Both David Linden and Christian Luscher have reported on the reward system operating behind neuroadaptation and development of tolerance to medications acting on reward pathways in the brain. Luscher and colleagues from University of Geneva specifically researched benzodiazepines as part of a larger project to identify the convergence point for all neurobiological pathways to drug addiction. Their findings endorse that this convergence occurs when dopamine surges with medication use cause a change in the synapses in dopamine-producing cells. They concluded that, as with opioids and cannabinoids, diazepam (Valium) and other benzodiazepines "take the brakes off the activity of dopamine-producing neurons".

And the importance of dopamine release in our lives? Linden describes how the dopamine neurotransmitter is tied up with both liking and wanting, (sleep, for instance), and even with salience, or emotional meaningfulness. He states "Part of what dopamine does seems to say, 'Here's something that is emotionally relevant and likely important for continued survival …so wake up and pay attention.' Dopamine also releases when there's uncertainty about potentially getting an imminent reward, so even before you take a sleep medication that expectancy for reward is creating dopamine release. Understandably, this makes it very difficult to come off a certain medication as tolerance builds (varying or reduced effectiveness) but the expectancy is strongly of reward.

CHAPTER 3   INSOMNIA & ANXIETY: THE EVOLUTION & IMPORTANCE OF ANXIETY TO HUMANS

Our brain's 2 oldest survival functions –functions of anxiety then and now - CBT cycle of anxiety - Understanding anxiety breathing physiology & calm breathing exercises - progressive muscle relaxation – jaw release – Worry & Rumination management.

All humans experience anxiety as a normal automatic emotion and physical response once a threat has been detected. Our sympathetic nervous system "fight or flight" response is governed by the oldest part of our brain, and has evolved over time to help us survive. This fight or flight response galvanises our body to flee (primarily) or fight (if cornered).

Our early ancestors were vulnerable in an environment with roaming predators and little protected habitation. A "hairtrigger" anxiety response and constant threat monitoring functioned to help them survive.

So our brains evolved to balance two basic survival functions:
1) to make us alert and physically ready to **fight or flee threats**, and
2) to **get us to sleep**

The balance is crucial because your brain and body would allow sleep in the past when it was safe to do so. This meant there had to be some leeway so that we early humans didn't drop down in overwhelming sleepiness as soon as darkness hit. That's where homeostatic drive fits in with your circadian drive.

FUNCTIONS OF ANXIETY THEN & NOW
Nowadays there is a mismatch between our ancient brain's vigilance for threat and our current environment. There are no longer roaming predators which would make light sleep functional, there are environmental stressors like work deadlines and road traffic jams. Social interactions are still somewhat threatening because now, as for our early ancestors, fitting in with a tribe is still important to our survival. But although social isolation can lead to loneliness and depression, we can still survive intact compared to the threat of social rejection by a tribe 30,000 years ago. Think of how much being ejected from a tribe would have affected secure sleep back then!

So just as early in our evolution, our capacity to detect and keep monitoring threats can help our survival. In modern life a moderate anxiety level can actually improve performance. Anxiety is only disruptive when it stops you from doing what you need or want to do. Let's say you're phobic about doctors and surgery: a certain amount of anxiety may galvanise you to take responsibility for your health, but become disruptive if it makes you avoid necessary surgery due to fear.

Think about how anxiety has been helpful for you in the past (eg, getting help early instead of waiting for it to get worse):
Anxiety was helpful for me when:
Now think about how anxiety has been unhelpful for you in the past:
Anxiety was unhelpful for me when:

The reasons some people are more anxious than others may include genetics (there is some evidence for an inherited "anxiety sensitivity" in some families); family history; early learning (eg observing parents' modelled anxiety responses) which led us to believe the world is more dangerous that it is, or we are not capable of coping with things; and more negative life events over which we felt we had little control.

Ultimately, it doesn't really matter why we are anxious, what matters more is that there are strategies to help us learn to manage anxiety that have been found to work after much research.

The three main features of the anxiety cycle are:
1) **thoughts and attention**, where your mind scans the environment for potential danger and decides 1) how likely it is a threat will happen, and 2) how bad/ severe it will be for us if it does (and also how capable we will be of coping and of managing the threat).

27

2) **Physical sensations** (fight/flight response) of increased heart rate, breathing rate, muscle tension, and importantly for sleep: core body temperature (an increased body temperature can stop us getting to or staying asleep). All these physical changes function to help us fight or run from danger and are compelled to happen as we detect threat).

3) **Escape/ safety behaviours** which include escape from a threat, avoiding an anticipated threat (could include thoughts, memories, body sensations, places, anxiety while we get through a feared situation, but longterm contribute to fear because we don't test our belief that the bad thing was avoided by our safety behaviour. In insomnia this is like being unable to calm ourselves enough to allow sleep. So we use sleep medication, feel relief at it successfully sedating us so we feel confident to fall asleep, but then worry more over time that we've lost the ability to get to sleep and need to rely on the medication to do the job.

This is the anxiety cycle that you can see underpins the insomnia cycle. The sleep medication is the safety-seeking behaviour we use in answer to the threat of losing sleep. It brings short term relief but more long term worry and rumination about the threat of poor sleep, keeping the anxiety symptoms and hypervigilance going (hypervigilance is the state of being highly alert and watchful for potential threats).

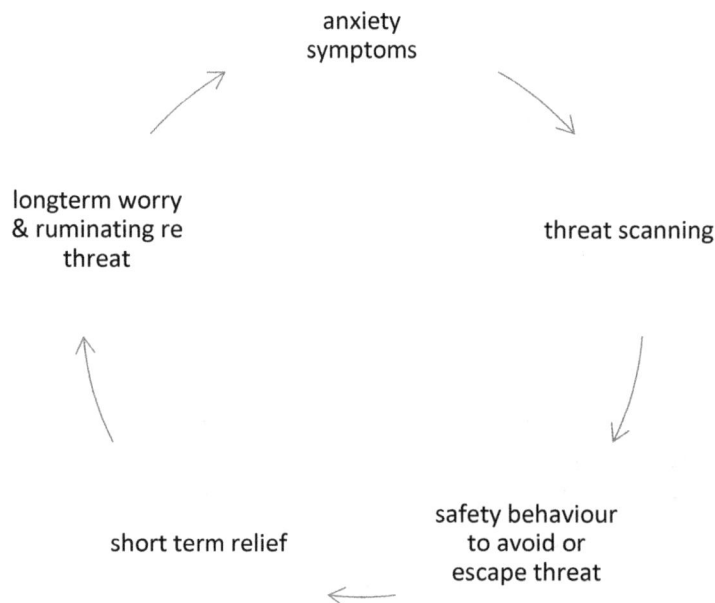

anxiety
symptoms

longterm worry
& ruminating re
threat

threat scanning

short term relief

safety behaviour
to avoid or
escape threat

Avoidance and escape, in bringing us short term relief, teach us the message that 1) the situation is dangerous and escape was necessary and 2) we aren't able to tolerate the anxiety feelings and sensations.

THE PRINCIPLES OF UNLEARNING ANXIETY

The way to unlearn anxiety is to
a) use new coping skills like slowed, controlled breathing and muscle relaxation to calm the nervous system, and
b) look at biases in our thinking that focus overly on our inability to cope, and on the uncontrollability and threat of the situation. That way we can:
c) gradually get back into a feared situation without ultimately needing safety behaviours that tell us we can't cope.

In insomnia, which is essentially performance anxiety about sleep, this means
a) learning some form of ongoing relaxation or meditation so we feel mastery at being able to calm our nervous system.
b) Then working on thoughts and expectations to catch biases in thinking that increase fear of not managing without medications.
c) then gradually getting back into the anxiety situation of allowing sleep to not be perfect or the solution to all our problems, while gradually reducing medication dose over time to test out managing sleep on our own.

This is not as easy as it sounds because the withdrawal symptoms as you reduce sleep medications will mimic the same anxiety symptoms you were trying to avoid in the first place. But the feelings of personal agency and self-mastery that come over time with keeping to a medication tapering schedule are a great antidote to the anxiety sensations because you feel you are more in control and have a concrete goal. It's bearable because the meaning you take from it is there's a purpose to any distress you're going through.

RELAXATION SKILLS to help you get through

We will start with understanding anxiety breathing physiology and how it affects our feelings; then introduce a calm breathing exercise, progressive muscle relaxation; and finally a jaw release exercise.

BREATHING AFFECTS FEELINGS

How we breathe affects the way we feel, in our senses and our emotions. When we are relaxed we naturally breathe lightly and slowly; but when we are anxious we breathe more heavily and quickly. This also works the other way: when we breathe heavily and quickly we can drive changes in our bloodstream that make us feel anxious, but when we breathe slowly and lightly we drive changes that make us feel calmer.

The rate and volume of our breathing affects the oxygen and carbon dioxide balance in our bloodstream. Inhaling takes in oxygen that is used by the body, creating the byproduct of carbon dioxide which we exhale. So when we are relaxed the levels of oxygen and carbon dioxide are balanced in the bloodstream.

INSOMNIA ANXIETY & BREATHING FASTER

When we are under threat we need more oxygenated blood to get to our major muscle groups. To do this we instinctively breathe faster and our heart rate speeds up when we believe danger is near (whether an external danger or an internal danger like being sleepless). This works well if we do in fact run or fight, because we will be appropriately using up the extra oxygen breathed in, and appropriately expelling the carbon dioxide breathed out. Which explains the agitation and desire to get up and pace at 2am if we can't sleep. Our brain and body are working together producing cortisol and adrenalin to mobilise us to escape from danger. And if our brain wants us to escape danger, at that point it doesn't want us to sleep. Of course the higher we value sleep the more sleeplessness seems dangerous.

Unfortunately this response uses up a lot of energy, so our core body temperature rises. Sleepiness is closely linked to reduced core body temperature. When our core body temperature rises with anxiety, then our heightened alertness is going to make it very difficult to get to sleep.

We could run around the block at 2am to use up the extra oxygen and appropriately expel the carbon dioxide. Exercise is a good way to deal with stress and overbreathing - during the day. At night a run would just increase our core body temperature and worsen our chances of resuming sleep. And unfortunately committing to staying motionless in bed when we're in anxious breathing will increase the imbalance of oxygen and carbon dioxide in our blood (a temporary change in the blood's pH called "respiratory alkalosis" which can feel like lightheadedness, tingling hands and feet and clamminess).

The good news is the brain will help out by self-regulating to slow the breathing and return the oxygen and carbon dioxide levels to normal or near-normal– it takes a lot of effort to keep fight-flight going if we are really panicking. And our threat-monitoring and "fight-flight" response also turns down once we believe that we're out of danger. This explains the attractiveness of the fast-acting sleep medications if we have begun to associate them with relief and calm that allows us to sleep. In fact the sleep medications *are* successful at slowing our breathing rate and volume (which can be dangerous if we forget and accidentally take too many pills). If we could test out what the brain does automatically to slow our breathing, by practising relaxing breathing skills daily, we might not need to turn to medication to slow our breathing and change our feelings.

Relaxed breathing exercises are pretty simple. Counting breaths is a good way for many people to steady their breathing rate *and* bat away racing thoughts. Try this one:

MINDFUL BREATHING EXERCISE

1) Lie down comfortably or sit with your back supported.
2) Close eyes if you feel comfortable and to reduce visual distraction(optional).
3) Breathe out first so you don't "top up" an existing lungful of air & end up overbreathing.

4) Then slightly pause after breathing out (not breath-holding, we want this to be smooth & fluid action).
5) Then breathe in through your nose lightly and steadily to a count of 4.
6) Then pause for a moment before breathing out steadily to a count of 4.
7) Repeat for 5 minutes at first, then try to increase to 10 minutes after a few weeks.
8) Expect feelings of frustration and doubt because your mind keeps racing - when you start training you won't likely concentrate on your breath for more than a few minutes. This *doesn't* mean you're doing it wrong or won't adapt to it! It takes Tibetan monks 40 years to learn the ability to centre and still their minds and be mindfully, nonjudgmentally, in the present moment. You won't get it overnight; no one will. Think of it as a training *process* and avoid being results-focused.
9) You can also record your breathing rate here (just count the number of breaths out in 30 seconds and double it to get your breaths per minute) as you practise daily (twice a day is ideal to start with). No pressure to slow your breathing effortly, just aim longer term for between 8-12 breaths per minute if lying in bed or sitting quietly.

day	mon	tue	wed	thur	fri	sat	sun
7am	Before	Before	Before	Before	Before	Before	Before
bpm	After	after	after	after	after	after	after
9pm	Before	before	before	before	before	before	before
bpm	After	after	after	after	after	after	after

JAW CLENCHING/TEETH GRINDING IN SLEEP:

If you tend to wake with TMJ soreness or aching and your dentist notes that you grind your teeth (a mouthguard while you sleep is a good investment!), try this jaw-clench release:

Jaw release if jaw clenching, with 3 steps:

A: pushing your tongue against the roof of your mouth relaxes the lower jaw muscles and temporo-mandibular joint (TMJ);

B: open your mouth slowly until wide without straining, close & repeat for 2 minutes.

C: place your closed fist under your chin pressed upwards lightly, then press your jaw downwards on closed fist without straining, for about 1 minute.

PROGRESSIVE MUSCLE RELAXATION

Try this muscle relaxation script to gain further awareness of when you are holding tension without realizing, and mastery in being able to relax your muscles when anxious or agitated.

Progressive muscle relaxation can help your mind and body relax through progressively tensing and relaxing muscle groups across your body. You just tense contract each muscle group for approximately 6 seconds (enough to feel some tightness but without straining), and then release the tension and notice 2 things: the difference between tension and relaxation, and the feeling of the muscle relaxing. If you notice pain or strong discomfort in any particular muscle group then you can choose to omit that step. As you do this exercise just attempt to visualize the muscles tensing and a relaxation "wave" flowing through them as you release that tension. And remember to keep breathing in and out steadily through the exercise- check in with your breath regularly to ensure you're not breath-holding. Now let's begin. You can record your voice on your phone and play it back with earphones, or record a friend reading this for you. Once you practise this every night as part of your bedtime routine, you can let go of the recording (which can initially help anchor your attention to your muscle groups) and just do the tense-relax scan on your own.

Begin by finding a comfortable position in a darkened room, either sitting with your back supported, or lying down, somewhere with no interruptions.

Bring your attention to focus on your internal senses, within your body. If you notice your mind wandering off, see this as a normal part of the process – it is the job of your brain to generate thoughts – and gently bring it back to the muscle group you are working on.

Take a slow, steady breath into your abdomen, hold for a count of 6 seconds while gently tensing your core abdominal muscles, then breathe out steadily and slowly as you release tension from the abdomen. Take another slow and steady breath in and as you breathe start to notice your abdomen rising while your chest and shoulders stay still. Again breathe down into the lower airways of your lungs, hold for a count of 6 seconds while gently tensing your core abdominal muscles, then breathe out steadily and slowly as you release tension from the abdomen. Feel your lower lung airways filling with refreshing air.

As you breathe out imagine the tension in your body releasing and flowing like a wave, out of your body.

And again breathe in.....and breathe out. Feel your body relaxing as it sinks with gravity and becomes heavier.

As you go through each step, remember to keep breathing and when you notice your mind wandering off, see this as normal and gently bring it back to the muscle group you are working on.

Now tense your forehead muscles by raising your eyebrows. Hold for 6 seconds. Then release the tension and notice the difference between the tension and the relaxation.

Pause for a few seconds.

Now frown and purse your lips, feeling the tense muscles of your brow and the tension in your lips and cheeks and jaw as you purse your lips. Hold for 6 seconds. Then release the tension and notice the difference between the tension and the relaxation in your brow, lips cheeks and jaw.

Now smile your biggest grin, feeling both mouth and cheek muscles tense. Hold for 6 seconds. Then release the tension and notice the difference between the tension and the relaxation in your lips, cheeks and jaw.

Pause for a few seconds.

Next, tense your eye muscles by squinting your eyes together tightly. Hold for 6 seconds, noticing the feelings of tension in these small muscles and surrounding muscles. Then release the tension and notice the difference between the tension and the relaxation in your eye muscles.

Pause for a few seconds.

Tilt your head back gently until you are looking at the ceiling. Hold for 6 seconds, noticing the feelings of tension in the neck muscles. Then release the tension and notice the difference between the tension and the relaxation in your neck muscles.

Pause for a few seconds.

Breathe in...and out.

Next, clench your hands into fists. Hold for 6 seconds, noticing the feelings of tension in the large and small muscles of the forearms and hands. Then release the tension and notice the difference between the tension and the relaxation in these muscles.

Pause for a few seconds.

Next, flex your biceps and feel the muscles contract. Hold for 6 seconds, noticing the feelings of tension in the large muscles of the arms. Then release the tension and notice the difference between the tension and the relaxation in these bicep muscles.

Pause for a few seconds.

Next, tense your tricep muscles by extending your arms out and locking your elbows, noticing the feelings of tension in the back of the arms. Then release the tension and notice the difference between the tension and the relaxation in these muscles.

Pause for a few seconds.

Next, tense your shoulder and back muscles by lifting your shoulders as if to touch your ears. Just feel the muscles contract. Hold for 6 seconds, noticing the feelings of tension in the large muscles of the back, shoulders, and arms. Then release the tension and notice the difference between the tension and the relaxation in these muscles.

Pause for a few seconds.

Next, tense your back muscles by lifting your shoulders back as if to touch your shoulder blades together. Just feel the muscles contract. Hold for 6 seconds, noticing the feelings of tension in the large muscles of the back, shoulders, and arms. Then release the tension and notice the difference between the tension and the relaxation in these muscles.

Pause for a few seconds.

Next, tense your chest muscles by deeply breathing in. Hold the breath for 6 seconds, noticing the feelings of tension in the muscles of the chest. Then release the tension and notice the difference between the tension and the relaxation in these chest muscles.

Pause for a few seconds.

Next, tense your stomach muscles by deeply sucking in these muscles. Hold the tension for 6 seconds, noticing these feelings of tension in the muscles stomach. Then release the tension and notice the difference between the tension and the relaxation in these muscles.

Pause for a few seconds.

Next, tense your lower back muscles by placing your hands on your hips and arching your lower back gently. Hold the tension for 6 seconds, then release the tension and notice the difference between the tension and the relaxation in the lower back muscles.

Notice the increased heaviness in your upper body as you let go of the tension and stress.

Pause for a few seconds.

Next, tense your buttock muscles and hold for 6 seconds, noticing the feelings of tension in these muscles. Then release the tension and notice the difference between the tension and the relaxation in these muscles.

Pause for a few seconds

Next, tense the thigh muscles by pressing your knees together, as if holding a book between them, and hold for 6 seconds, noticing the feelings of tension in these thigh muscles. Then release the tension and notice the difference between the tension and the relaxation in these muscles.

Pause for a few seconds.

Now tense the muscles in your feet, pulling your toes towards you and feeling the tension in your shins. Hold for 6 seconds, noticing the feelings of tension in these feet, ankle and shin muscles. Then release the tension and notice the difference between the tension and the relaxation in these muscles.

Pause for a few seconds.

Now tense the muscles under your feet, pointing your toes away with legs straight and feeling the tension in your calves. Hold for 6 seconds, noticing the feelings of tension in these feet, ankle and calf muscles. Then release the tension and notice the difference between the tension and the relaxation in these muscles.

Pause for a few seconds.

Visualise now a wave of relaxation spreading gradually throughout your body, from the top of your head and going down to your feet.

Feel the heaviness of your muscles across your body. Take this relaxed feeling with you into bed and just let sleep happen, without effort or control.

day	mon	tue	wed	thur	fri	sat	sun
7am	Before	Before	Before	Before	Before	Before	Before
Tension level/10	After	after	after	after	after	after	after
9pm	Before	before	before	before	before	before	before
Tension level/10	After	after	after	after	after	after	after

CHAPTER 4 OUR SLEEP PROCESSES
The homeostatic and circadian drives that look after our sleep: the tools in this program to get sleep back on track. - The normal circadian sleep wake cycle and when things go off-track. -Delayed or advanced circadian rhythm sleep-wake disorders.

There are two primary mechanisms driving our sleep–wake cycle: One process follows a "circa diem" or circadian rhythm and is independent of sleeping and waking. The other process (the homeostatic drive process) depends on sleep-wake actions: sleepiness dissipates during sleep and rises continuously during wakefulness.

1) <u>HOMEOSTATIC DRIVE</u>, or 'sleep pressure', ie need or drive for sleep. The longer we're awake, the longer our sleep deprivation, the greater the pressure. This is how our homeostatic drive works if we have a regular 10pm-6am sleep schedule daily. Along with the increasing pressure to sleep that builds over a day is a sleep-regulating substance in the brain called adenosine. Adenosine is created during our day's waking hours, as a natural byproduct of burning through our internal energy supplies. It's the core of an energy-storing molecule which powers most of the biochemical reactions inside cells.

Here's our homeostatic drive and associated adenosine buildup over a regular sleep-wake pattern:

Regular 8 hour sleep - wake pattern

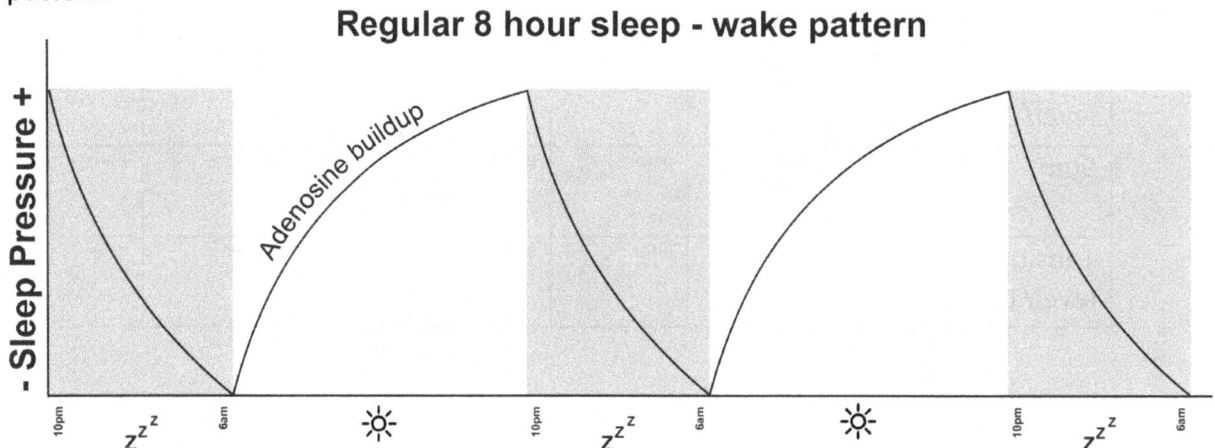

Now here's what happens to our homeostatic sleep pressure if we miss a night's sleep:
One night's sleep missed

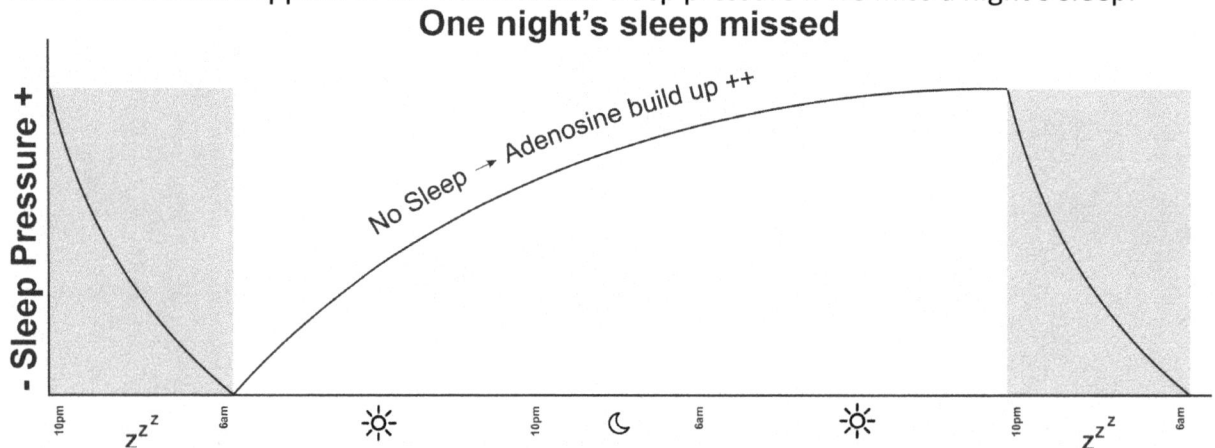

As you can see adenosine buildup reflects growing sleep pressure over our waking hours. If we miss out on a night's sleep or only have 2-3 hours sleep one night, adenosine will continue to accumulate in the cerebrospinal fluid and homeostatic drive will continue to build until we sleep. High levels of adenosine lead to sleepiness, so you can think of adenosine as a "sleep-inducer". You can dampen the sleepiness by blocking the adenosine receptors with caffeine, but only temporarily, and not for a guaranteed period of time. Which is why using caffeine to prevent microsleeps while driving is a fraught business.

2) CIRCADIAN drive: this is our internal, biological clock, generated from a wakeup clock in our brain called the suprachiasmatic nucleus (SCN). Morning sunlight entering the eye (even through closed eyelids) travels along the retinal nerve, hits the SCN, and resets the circadian rhythm. The SCN then turns down melatonin sleep hormone production.

The SCN also helps us with sleep onset at night. It connects with the pineal gland, which releases melatonin as darkness falls. The SCN ensures melatonin levels rise during the night and fall towards dawn. This will be explained in further detail later in this book.

SUNLIGHT AND SEROTONIN

We really are intrinsically "solar-powered" creatures: sunlight has the power to not only re-set our circadian rhythm each morning but also "re-set" or improve our mood, by optimising our serotonin neurotransmission. Three interrelated hormones involved in our sleep cycle are tryptophan, melatonin and serotonin. Tryptophan is an amino acid that produces Serotonin. Serotonin is light-sensitive, regulates sleep, calms your central nervous system, and is converted by your pineal gland into melatonin. As the evening draws into darkness, the body's serotonin levels rise and melatonin is released to start the natural sleep cycle, just as core body temperature drops overnight. This is shown in the picture below (inspired by Flinders University's sleep specialist Leon Lack).

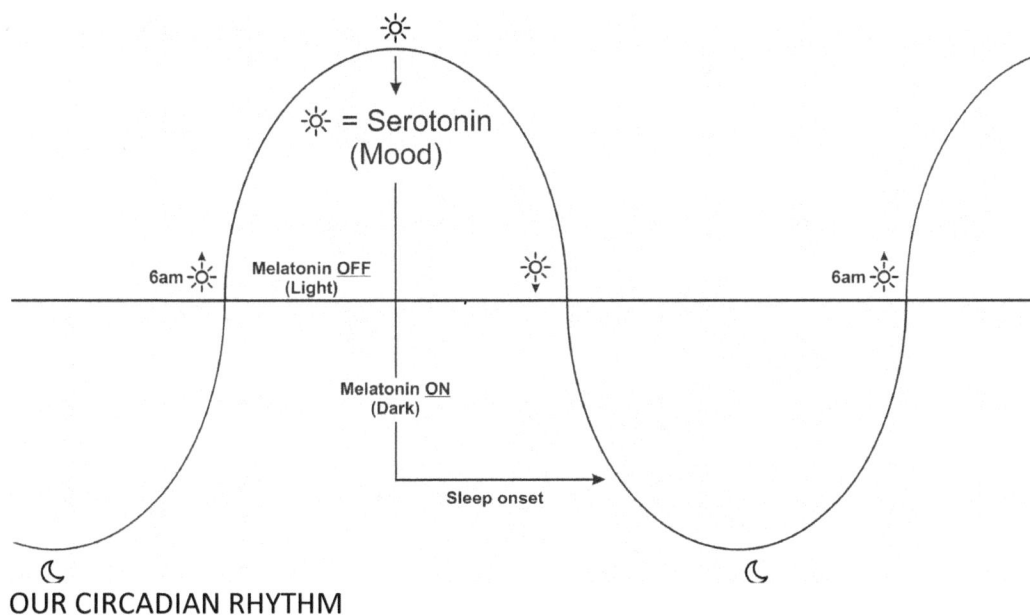

OUR CIRCADIAN RHYTHM

The circadian rhythm and homeostatic sleep pressure work together to converge naturally after darkness falls, assuming we have spent the sunlight hours awake and alert (not dozing). With the help of melatonin production we get sleep onset, and with the accumulated pressure of homeostatic drive, we go down into deep sleep within 30 to 40 minutes. The deep sleep is always in the first half of the night, as a direct result of the accumulated adenosine accumulating throughout the day's waking hours (see the sleep stages graph in this chapter).

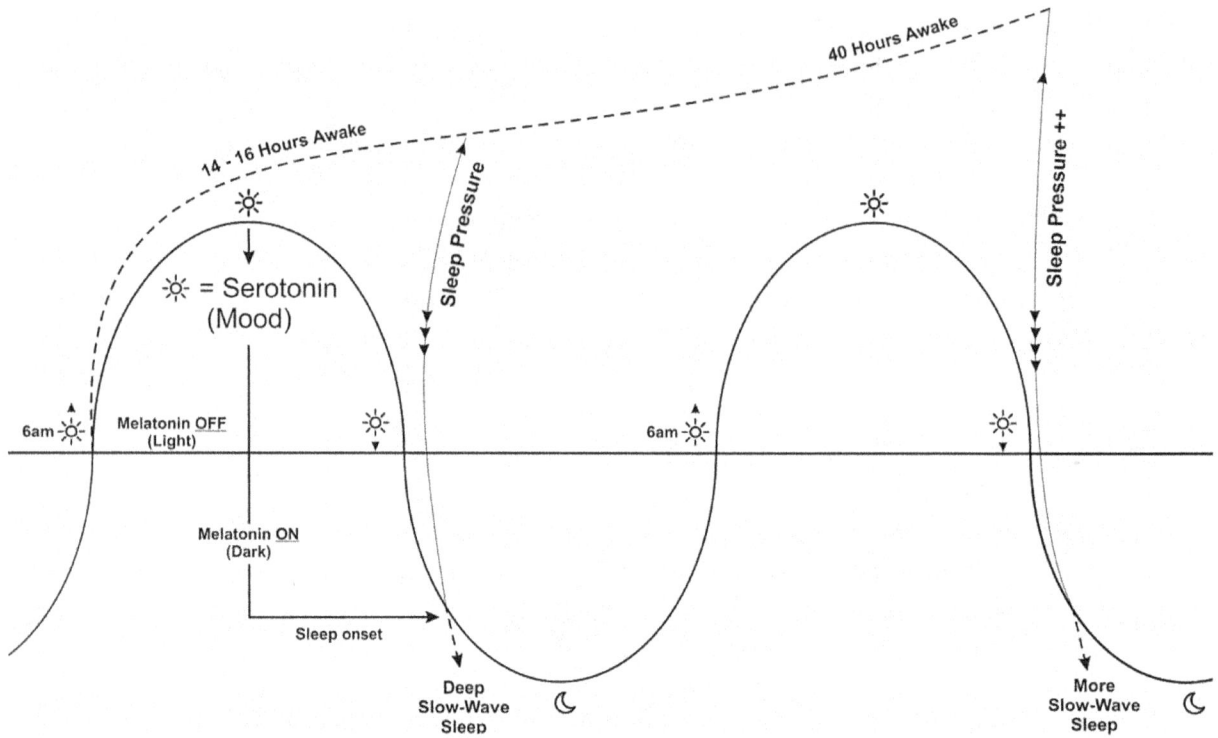

14 - 16 Hours Awake

40 Hours Awake

Sleep Pressure

Sleep Pressure ++

☀ = Serotonin
(Mood)

6am ☀   Melatonin OFF
(Light)

Melatonin ON
(Dark)

Sleep onset

Deep
Slow-Wave
Sleep

6am ☀

More
Slow-Wave
Sleep

HOW OUR CIRCADIAN RHYTHM AND HOMEOSTATIC DRIVE WORK TOGETHER

AWAKE   ASLEEP   AWAKE

Core Body Temperature

Sleepiness

Minimum Core
Temp

Melatonin - Sleep Hormone

| 8am | 10am | | 2pm | 4pm | 6pm | 8pm | 10pm | | 2am | 4am | 6am | 8am | 10am | | 2pm |
| | | Midday | | | | | | Midnight | | | | | | Midday | |

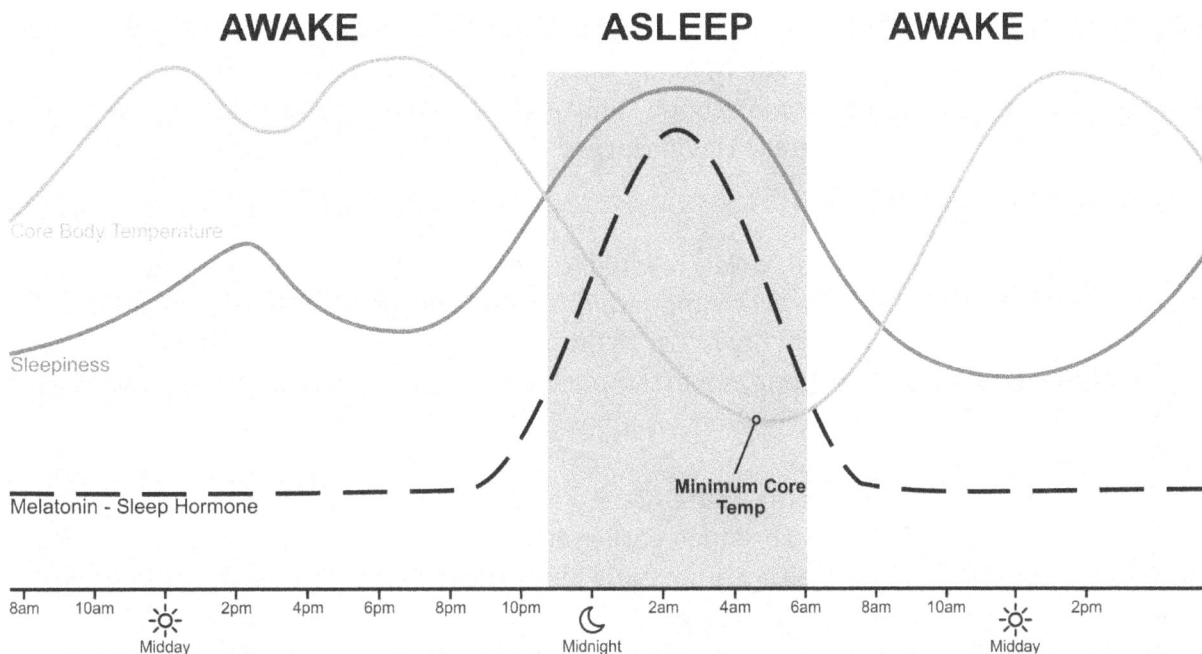

CORE BODY TEMPERATURE, SLEEPINESS FLUCTUATIONS AND MELATONIN PRODUCTION

Our circadian rhythm keeps us in rhythm with our natural environment, working with the sun's rise and fall, light and dark. Normal sleep is regulated by the rotation of the earth and daylight, so is "circular" and around 24 hours for a full sleep and wake cycle. Within this cycle there are also "ultradian" rhythms which are temperature fluctuations and relative sleepiness (and alertness), that go up and down during the day and night. So, there are drowsiness/alertness cycles within the 24-hour drowsiness/alertness cycle). This short drop in core body temperature after lunch accounts for that post-lunch, early afternoon sleepiness. The "second wind" or burst of energy that insomnia sufferers report in the late afternoon or early evening, after a day of fatigue, coincides with the increase in core body temperature before the final drop heralding sleep onset.

LARKS VS OWLS
There are normal differences (delays or advances) in the periods in which we sleep compared to other people. Some people have the chronobiology of larks, which means they wake and rise early and fall asleep early in the night; other people have the chronobiology of owls, meaning they tend to wake and rise later in the morning and feel sleepy later at night. This only becomes a problem when there is ongoing sleep disruption due to a mismatch between our own natural waking and our social/ work/study requirements. And this ongoing sleep disruption can lead to real distress and social or work impairment, due to insomnia or excessive daytime sleepiness arising from the sleep deprivation (for example, in adolescents who fall asleep at 3am after being on electronic devices, and then need to wake for school at 7am – over time this leads to real sleep deprivation).

DELAYED CIRCADIAN SLEEP-WAKE DISORDER & SLEEP DEPRIVATION
It's very disruptive if an owl tendency becomes delayed sleep phase disorder, because we are now talking about very real sleep deprivation. This means delayed sleep onset and waking times, that don't match up with school or workplace start times, and real *inability* to sleep and be awake at times that help functioning at work, university or school. This entails

39

students or workers getting up with multiple alarms ringing, at their core body temperature minimum, with slowed thinking and reaction time because their brain wants them to be asleep for a few more hours. Some schools, universities and colleges are leaning toward later start times to accommodate this widespread late-waking, and students are reporting improved grades since the change.

I know several clients – bilingual, luckily – who moved to adjacent Asian countries 3 - 4 hours behind Australian time to accommodate their delayed circadian sleep-wake difficulty. This didn't always work longterm however, as after initial success in getting to work on time they adapted to the new time zone; several months later they were again falling asleep at 2-3am and having difficulty rising for work.

ADVANCED CIRCADIAN SLEEP-WAKE DISORDER
These are people with advanced or much earlier night-time sleep onset and earlier waking times. It's about falling asleep easily quite early in the night – often around 8-9pm when other people are just starting to socialise, watch films, etc. It also means waking in the early hours of the morning once the brain has fully met the person's sleep needs. For older people waking early in the morning after a full sleep can be lonely and distressing thinking everyone else is sleeping soundly and will be for another 3 hours. These people will describe a simple inability to stay awake after 9pm even though they miss having active social lives at night.
The advanced sleep phase type doesn't generally have such a cost as the delayed type; there is at least plenty of opportunity for sleep and not functional impairment from sleep deprivation. Apologies to those of you sleeping from 9pm who disagree, but people with Delayed sleep-wake cycles actually lose the *opportunity* to sleep further. Advanced sleep-wake cycle people have the opportunity to sleep but not the *ability* to sleep longer into the morning.

IRREGULAR SLEEP-WAKE PATTERNS
There are also irregular sleep-wake types where people have variable sleep-wake periods or non-24-hour sleep-wake type (which is a pattern of sleeping and waking not synchronised or anchored to 24 hours but consistently drifting forward in time). Circadian sleep wake disorders can hurt shift workers hard, if they have nonconventional work hours that keep shifting. If a worker is flying in-flying out of a remote worksite they may adjust well enough to shift work in the second half of the work week. But upon flying home for even a weekend almost everyone will revert back to a day waking and night-sleeping pattern to fit in with their families and friends' sleep-wake cycles.

SLEEP CYCLES AND SLEEP STAGES
Throughout the night's sleep, we move in and out of various sleep stages in approximately 90 minute cycles (of which we need about 4 or 5 to get maximum benefit from sleep). During these sleep cycles we spend time in Rapid Eye Movement (REM, or dream) sleep and NonREM sleep (which includes deep and light sleep stages).

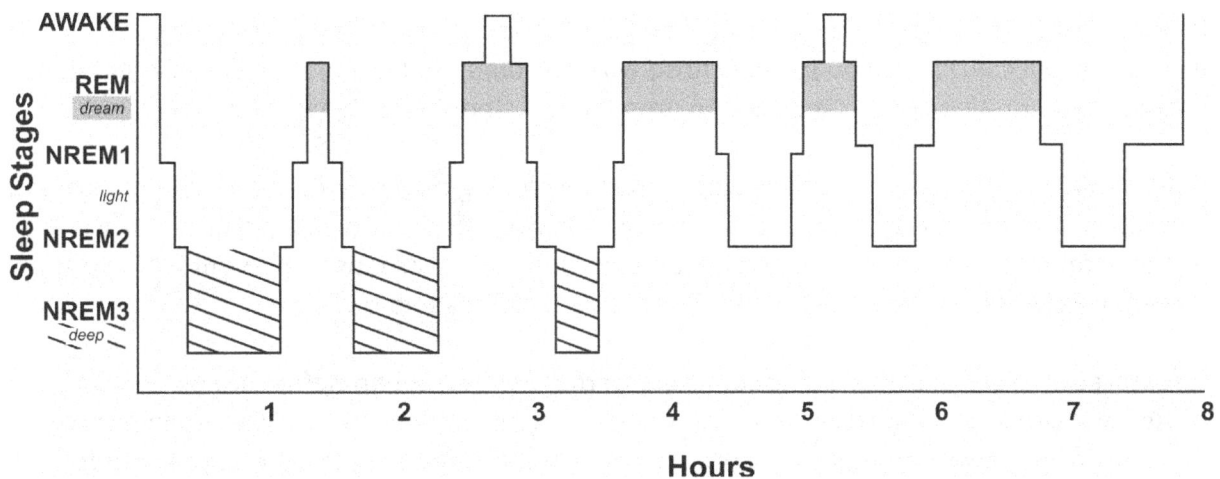

OUR SLEEP STAGES

NREM STAGE 1 is a transition period between wakefulness and sleep lasting about 5-10 minutes, during which the brain transitions from producing nonsynchronized beta and gamma brain waves (representing wakeful state frequency waves) to slower, more synchronized alpha waves, to high amplitude theta waves (very slow brain waves). If a person is woken during this stage, they may report that they weren't really asleep.

NREM STAGE 2 is the threshold into deeper sleep, where people are less aware of their surroundings and where core body temperature drops and heart rate slows. This stage lasts around 20 minutes, and is where the brain starts producing sleep spindles (rapid, rhythmic brain wave activity). About 50% of total sleep is spent in NREM stage 2.

NREM STAGE 3 is deep, slow-wave sleep, where muscles relax, blood pressure and breathing rate drop, cell and tissue repair occur, and human growth hormone is produced, and the glymphatic system in the brain flushes byproducts of energy expenditure accumulated during the day's wakefulness. Nava Zisapel, neuroscientist at Tel Aviv University, has described the brain's glymphatic system as an efficient "sewerage" system, in which the space between the brain cells widens and is "flushed out" in deep sleep.

Previously divided into stages 3 and 4, Stage 3 features slow brain waves called delta waves and is where people become generally unresponsive to noises or activity in the environment. It is very hard to wake someone from deep sleep, and the confusion and grogginess or "sleep inertia" is severe if someone is forced to wake from deep sleep. Deep, slow-wave sleep is directly linked to homeostatic drive and adenosine buildup. Essentially the pressure to sleep building up during the day is pressure to go into deep non-REM sleep.

Within around 30 minutes of going to sleep we descend into slow-wave sleep (which is why we try to restrict afternoon naps to under 30 minutes). So we always experience Slow-Wave Sleep or deep sleep during first half of the night – it is strongly related to the amount of time we have spent awake during the day. Then we spend more time in REM/dream sleep and light sleep in the second half of the night.

If we miss out on a night's sleep or only have a 2-3 hours sleep, sleep pressure and adenosine will continue to build over those waking hours, and the brain will self-regulate to ensure the deep sleep needs increase in urgency and sleepiness signals grow stronger.

REM Rapid Eye Movement sleep is where most dreaming occurs, with rapid eye movement, increased respiration rate, and increased brain activity, yet paradoxically muscle tone is lost as the involuntary muscles relax and become immobilised (perhaps to prevent acting out of dreams). REM sleep constitutes about 20 percent of total sleep time.

It features involves memory consolidation, filtering out non-meaningful data or "white noise" and consolidating meaningful material in long term memory. REM sleep in particular helps us form new memories which then helps us learn. Sleep prescription medications which disrupt laying down of episodic memory (so we less easily recall waking periods at night) can therefore affect new learning. REM sleep is also important for emotion regulation; if we miss a night's sleep we will generally notice our emotions are harder to manage or quiet.

CHAPTER 5   ATTENTION PROCESSES IN INSOMNIA.

Attention and insomnia. Scanning for noise threats creates more vigilance, worry and rumination, and sleeplessness. How tinnitus research helps insomnia treatment. Relaxation & breathing skills engage attention and increase acceptance and calm.

Your brain, your central nervous system and your attention processes work together to warn you about things going wrong. This chapter looks at over-attention in insomnia to the threat of sleep loss, which leads to strong emotion responses and central nervous system activation to fight or flee the threat. The way threat monitoring works in tinnitus is a good example of how insomnia hypervigilance starts up and keeps going. And also how attention biases start up and link in with nervous system hyperalertness. Tinnitus treatment also uses Attention Training habituation (or as Pavlov called it "extinction of orientation reaction" in his famous dog studies) from which we can borrow for insomnia treatment.

Why tinnitus treatment? Understandably, you may think there are many distractions that can grab the attention and threaten a night's sleep. Visual distractions (like a neon light flashing outside the bedroom window) and aggravating textures or surfaces. Because even if people can wear eyemasks and buy new sleep linen or mattresses, it's very difficult to turn off attention to unwanted and uncontrollable environmental noises. Freedman and colleagues defined noise as "unwanted sounds that could have negative psychological and physiological effects." In their studies of ICU's (intensive care units) on environmental noise sleep disruption effects they found widespread patient beliefs that ICU sleep quality was significantly poorer than baseline sleep at home because of such uncontrollable noise.

Uncontrollability of noise is an important factor in generating hyperacute (very acute) hearing and fight-flight nervous system response; the response is the same in insomnia as it is in tinnitus. Irritant sounds take on threat meaning and set up a conditioned nervous system and emotional response. That gets practised over and over again, until we're stuck in hypervigilance, *seeking* out irritating sounds as soon as our heads hit the pillow.

NOISES THAT AFFECT MY SLEEP (record emotion intensity out of 10 next to each)	
Controllable noises:	**Uncontrollable noises:**
Irritation/anxiety intensity /10	**Irritation/anxiety intensity /10**

HOW TINNITUS RESEARCH CAN HELP OVERCOME INSOMNIA
Tinnitus is equivalent to a phantom auditory sensation. It is the perception of sound (hissing, ringing, buzzing, static, cicadas, etc) resulting from nervous system activation without any corresponding mechanical vibrations in the cochlea, and no external stimulation of any kind.

Tinnitus has been a problem for humans for thousands of years, and different treatments tried without consistent success. It affects about 17%- 30% of the population depending on how it is assessed and measured in a particular country. So tinnitus perception is common - but not everyone with tinnitus is suffering with it. It's an interesting fact that there is no difference between tinnitus "experiencing" and "suffering" groups in tinnitus loudness pitch.

TINNITUS SUFFERING LIES WITH THE EMOTION & FIGHT/FLIGHT BRAIN SYSTEMS
It is not the brain's auditory system that is responsible for tinnitus severity and perceived suffering but other brain systems – the limbic system (controls our emotions) and the autonomic nervous system (controlling automatic functions like heart and breathing rate, muscle tone, hormones, digestion, the "fight or flight" response generally).

TINNITUS AND SLEEP DISTURBANCE LINKS
Around 50% of people with tinnitus have disturbed sleep. Problem tinnitus generates high levels of central nervous system fight-flight activation/alertness all through the day and night. Also the brain's hearing centre is very active at a subconscious level during sleep, and the hearing and emotion (limbic) systems are closely connected at this level. During the light sleep stages and upon waking during the night, attention will immediately turn to tinnitus signals, which will be perceived as loud relative to the quiet background sounds at night. This threat perception will cause further nervous system fight-flight activation, and further emotional reactivity. Plus the increased risk of depression due to both sleep disturbance as well as ongoing problems with attention, concentration and activities done in quiet environments.

TINNITUS AND CONDITIONED NEGATIVE ASSOCIATIONS
The tinnitus signal itself causes no harm, and suffering only develops when it becomes associated with something negative and creates strong limbic (emotional) and autonomic (fight or flight) nervous system reactions. Once tinnitus acquires negative associations it triggers constant monitoring. How do the negative associations build? If your tinnitus signal causes strong emotional distress, you will start up a conditioned reflex causing your brain's hearing centre to keep strongly activating your emotion and fight-flight systems. The feedback loop between the emotion and fight-flight systems strengthens to keep your attention "seeking out" the threatening noise.

HOW HYPERACUTE HEARING IN INSOMNIA FITS IN
This is just like hyperacute hearing in insomnia. The smallest sound, whether constant or intermittent, gets appraised as threatening, activates your emotion system and with it the fight-flight system. The negative association starts building and becomes a conditioned reflex to keep your brain's hearing centre activating your (frustrated, anxious) emotion and

fight-flight responses. The result: increased core body temperature and threat monitoring – and sleep disturbance.

NATURALLY "GETTING USED TO" THREATENING SOUNDS
Jastreboff and Hazell (2008) write about the fact that more than ¾ of people who experience tinnitus "habituate" naturally to it. "Habituation" just means the nervous system is adapting to or "getting used to" an initially threatening noise. Because of the way our brains evolved to notice new and unfamiliar objects and events, we detect and monitor unfamiliar potential "threats", but start to ignore them when they become familiar or routine, and no longer threatening. As this happens not only our attention fades, but our emotion (limbic) system response reduces and our nervous system calms down with it.

When this happens in tinnitus, over time these people are no longer aware of the tinnitus signal unless they consciously focus attention on it. Habituation starts happening naturally, as the nervous system reduces its reaction with the repeated unchanging signal. Then as the tinnitus signal is presented repeatedly without being followed by any fight-flight or strong emotional response the attention just fades away. There's no need to keep monitoring for threats. It's literally like "nothing to see here folks, might as well go home".

This is especially important for insomnia sufferers with hyperacute hearing, the people who wake at sounds that others might easily ignore. Their emotion and fight-flight brain systems fire up as they judge the sound threatening, and their attention stays on to keep monitoring the threat.

HABITUATION TO OVERCOME FIGHT-FLIGHT ANXIETY RESPONSE
To get habituation going, we need to try 2 things in insomnia:
One is to accept: that these are the oldest parts of our brain working to assess if a sound is threatening and to keep us from danger. Our brain is compelled to do this and keep us awake if there's something we judge threatening. We can't get angry at it; it's not "broken", it's working perfectly well doing its most basic survival task.

Two, because of the above, we would need to communicate to our brain compelling evidence that we are not under threat if we want it to start to ignore the sounds. Just pretending there's no threat won't work with the brain – our belief strength and emotion intensity is going to shout louder than any attempts at "positive" self-talk. If we really believe - and *care* – that we're going to get sick or sacked because this noise is stopping our sleep we won't be able to talk ourselves into thinking or caring otherwise. We would need to have real evidence that we're not in danger. That's why it's important to go through the beliefs and expectations chapter and work on catching attention and thinking biases. A bias for catastrophizing in our thinking will definitely drive ongoing threat monitoring around sleep.

WHAT I HAVE DONE TO COPE WITH NOISES THAT AFFECT MY SLEEP (record success level out of 10 next to each)	
Controllable noises:	Uncontrollable noises:
Coping ability /10	Coping ability /10

HOW SELECTIVE PERCEPTION MAKES NOISE A PROBLEM

If we judge a new sound as unimportant it will not activate the emotion and fight/flight systems. Even with the sound repeating, the higher brain function/cortical areas controlling sound awareness will block it and we won't be aware of it. This is called **habituation of perception.** The sound no longer induces the anxious flight/flight reaction (**habituation of reaction**).

However, if a sound is familiar but important (to our safety), ie threatening, its repeated appearance results in strong limbic/emotion and fight/flight reactions *every* time we are exposed to it. This is called "hyperacuity", an extreme reaction to the threat sound.

Selective perception is an important attention mechanism, and an important brain limitation: only one task can occupy our focus of attention at any given time. We cannot perform more than one task that requires full attention at the same time. We solve it by rapidly switching from one attention focus to another, and performing other tasks automatically. For example, car driving: our brain continuously does complex tasks automatically while blocking most sensory information from reaching our cortical awareness. This "peak automaticity" lets us arrive at a familiar destination with little memory of the drive.

TREATING HYPERACUITY

In summary, once we link an incoming signal with something negative (fear or frustration), we can't remove this link as its part of a conditioned reflex. We have no way to directly control the reflexive emotional or fight/flight reactions as these are necessary for survival. A conditioned reflex cannot be altered by conscious thoughts alone.

Tinnitus severity is decided by nervous system and emotional/limbic system, which together determine whether we are threatened and "suffering" or instead just "experiencing" tinnitus. Tinnitus severity is not about the loudness of the tinnitus sound but how your emotion system and central nervous system react to it. The more threatening you find the sound, the more your central nervous system is involuntarily in fight or flight, and the more your hearing sense *searches* for the sound. Your nervous and limbic systems decide whether you are suffering, or just experiencing tinnitus sounds.

That's why anti-anxiety medication seems to work so well for hyperacuity – in both tinnitus and insomnia. It's quieting your central nervous system generally, not targeting your tinnitus sounds or insomnia noise-hearing. But it's a mistake to use anti-anxiety medications like valium or alcohol to quiet your fight-flight and reduce your tinnitus reactivity. When the medication or alcohol sedating effects wear off your brain's hearing centre will still be searching for the sound and threatened by it. You won't have *desensitized* to the sound. And that leads to panic once people develop tolerance to the sedative medication, (it no longer controls anxiety symptoms effectively). Once a person is suffering "hyperacuity" - is extremely reactive to the threatening sound - it's very difficult to turn down the emotional and fight-flight response.

A SOUND ENRICHMENT PROGRAM

In tinnitus we react not to the absolute strength of a sound but its *relative strength compared with background sound*. This works the same for all senses: a candle appears very bright in dark room but is almost invisible in broad daylight. In silence, tinnitus is the only sound present and will perk up your auditory system's attentional focus. When background sound is at a low level, our hearing becomes more acute than when higher background sound levels exist. So if you have tinnitus you can use white noise to mask the tinnitus, and then grow used to it.

Avoiding silence and instead seeking *continuous background sounds*, is the core treatment in tinnitus and reduces hyperacuity of your attention to the sound. So the goal of attention training in hyperacuity treatment is *desensitizing the auditory system* by systematic exposure to a variety of sounds, called an "enriching program". Through enriching background sounds, and amplifying this enriched, non-aversive sound we get habituation of reaction (no further "high alert" nervous system or emotional response) and habituation of perception (we are no longer aware of the repellent sound, except when we focus attention on it).

A tinnitus retraining program focuses on practising "enrichment" of the auditory background, keeping a constant background level of sound that is not annoying or attention-triggering. It means learning that background sound is helpful in desensitizing to the tinnitus while silence is unhelpful, and so actively avoiding silence.

So how can this help insomnia sufferers? If a person with insomnia has hyperacute hearing and threat monitoring of the smallest sounds then the desensitization treatment to insomnia hyperacuity is the same as desensitization to tinnitus.

NOISE-MASKING TO CALM THE NERVOUS SYSTEM

The director of sleep medicine at Canyon Ranch in Tucson, Arizona, Param Dedhia, suggests you can affect your (emotional) response to a loud sound with auditory masking (via a noise machine). What kind of noise machine? White-noise generators are a burgeoning industry of mechanical and digital devices, apps and websites, and subscribable playlists. All seek to market white noise of various descriptions. There are DIY white-noise solutions for tinnitus and insomnia sufferers (such as using a box cutter to roughen box fan blades).

Engineers identified white noise back in the 1920s, using it as a test signal because it's "the sum of all the audible frequencies in equal proportion in a single sound. It's so named because of its analogy to light, which turns white when all visible frequencies are summed up into a single beam" according to Stephane Pigeon, a Belgian electrical engineer who developed Mynoise.net, an online sound generator.

Sample "enrichment" programs could include "white noise" (eg Dohm-like) machines, humidifiers, fans and other devices. Babies are used to and comforted by the maternal circulatory system and womb, sleeping better accompanied by a device that mimics those familiar whooshing sounds (like the washing machine or white noise devices).

MEANING-MAKING TO CALM THE NERVOUS SYSTEM

Noise is subjective and very individual: Some people are soothed by a partner's snoring because of the meaning it holds for them (closeness). Other people are irritated by it, especially as it is very difficult to mask (inescapably near your ears if you're in the same bed) and the gasps are threatening (hold meaning of partner's ill health if apnoeic periods happen and breathing stops for a period) and arrive unpredictably (again if breathing stops – apnoea – you are actively listening for the next gasp).

Pigeon suggests convincing ourselves that the snoring reflects something good or meaningful (like relationship closeness) but understandably this will be a tough ask for most. There is increasing real estate data showing Australian retirement-age couples are no longer downsizing the family home for something smaller. Or they are seeking larger apartments with spare bedrooms. Around 80% of the insomnia patients I see who are in a relationship report now relying on the spare bedroom refuge for sleep-safeguarding – whether or not they use it every night. The spare bedroom becomes a backup, "rabbit's foot" for ensuring coping in insomnia.

It highlights that uncontrollability is a significant factor; if we can find "a way around" so that we feel we have some control over the noise and make it "our own" then we may feel personal agency and mastery, so then we will cope better and habituate more easily to the sound. To help, there are acoustic and noise-abatement experts who design white noise programs to play on home speakers that will be tuned to block a pure tone (any sound that has a specific and constant musical pitch, like building construction sounds). Or we can start from the internal mastery angle, using relaxation and meditation daily to calm the nervous system. A quietened nervous system means less reacting to and hypervigilance around outside noises we can't control.

WHAT I CAN TRY IN MY SOUND ENRICHMENT PROGRAM TO CHANGE THE MEANING OR THREAT VALUE OF NOISES AFFECTING MY SLEEP (record success level out of 10 next to each at 3 week review)	
Controllable/uncontrollable noises:	Sound enrichment ideas:
Success level /10	Success level /10

A final word on relying on only TV as your sound enrichment program, to engage your attention in insomnia. It doesn't seem like a bad idea, but TV has variable noise levels (ad breaks) and variable light, which will perk your nervous system up as your attention catches on something interesting, and your frontal lobe becomes engaged in a way that pushes sleep away.

CHAPTER 6   THE ESSENTIAL HABITS AND ACTIONS TO GET SLEEP BACK ON TRACK

The effective interventions. Essential morning, evening and night-time actions to get sleep back on track and let the brain get on with its sleep regulation job.

The American College of Physicians (ACP) recommends that all adult insomnia patients receive cognitive behavioural therapy for insomnia (CBT-I) as the initial treatment for chronic insomnia disorder (strong recommendation, moderate-quality evidence). The American Academy of Sleep Medicine (AASM) ranks treatments based on degree of clinical certainty of effectiveness. The AASM rankings of psychological sleep interventions state:

- Stimulus control therapy, targeting behaviours incompatible with sleep & retraining associating bed with sleep, has a "High degree of clinical certainty";
- Progressive muscle relaxation, a "moderate degree of clinical certainty... probably efficacious";
- Sleep hygiene education: "insufficient evidence as a single therapy"

The Insomnia CBT program here contains all the psychological sleep interventions with the highest clinical certainty ratings: it is the behaviour change experiments that have the strongest effectiveness in helping people unlearn their habitual insomnia-reinforcing actions. These experiments are designed to help us reassociate our beds with sleep, using conditioning processes and habit formation principles to help people train out of insomnia.

LETSLEEPHAPPEN CORE UNLEARNING INSOMNIA ACTIONS & LEARNING OBJECTIVES
The essential actions needed to regulate your sleep-wake cycle and pave the way to trust and confidence in your sleep are these (with the learning objectives of each):

MORNING AND DAYTIME ACTIONS
1. Same waking and rising time daily (to align with the sun rising, & to reset sleep wake schedule in accord with the body's internal circadian rhythms)
2. Early morning sunlight (to turn off melatonin sleep hormone production and reset your circadian rhythm, because 82% of your body's tissues have a circadian rhythm governed by light and dark. Also to improve your mood).
3. If natural waking time is more than 4 hours after dawn, set an alarm for the natural waking time & get exposure to bright light. Then set alarm and get up 30 minutes earlier for 1+ hour sunlight exposure on each subsequent day until goal waking & rising time is achieved (to overcome sleep onset difficulties and a delayed sleep-wake cycle). If natural waking time is 3 hours before dawn use bright light and socializing (but not stimulants) in the evenings to train the sleep forward (to change an advanced sleep-wake cycle).
4. Avoid naps during the daytime if you have current insomnia, to build up homeostatic pressure over the day's waking hours.

5. Energetic exercise early in the day but only a gentle stroll after 5pm (for general health, mood and sleep quality, muscle relaxation, and to accentuate the body's natural temperature cooling and nervous system calming before bed)

NIGHT-TIME ACTIONS

1. Core body temperature and sleep: avoid stimulants (nicotine, caffeine) before bed. Lifestyle and dietary triggers to insomnia, as part of basic sleep "hygiene" – practices to assist sleep regularity. Also to learn about your central nervous system's sympathetic vs parasympathetic responses).

2. Build a sleep-friendly bedroom environment: Complete or near-complete darkness, cooler ambient temperature, reduced noise & no daytime activities in bed (to calm nervous system and condition sleepiness to the bed).

3. Train a regular bedtime wind-down ritual (strengthening conditioned associations between your bed and sleepiness using associative learning principles)

4. Go to bed only when sleepy (to reduce your chances of bed being associated with wakefulness).

5. Avoid hypnotic substances pre-bedtime (alcohol, prescription sleep medications) if you are not already on them, but if currently dependent on sleep medications don't stop suddenly. Work with your prescriber to establish a tapering regime to reduce alongside InsomniaCBT (to understand attributing sleep to substances, and preparedness to learn sleep habits & calm nervous system on one's own vs depend on sedative and hypnotic medications to get to sleep).

6. Get out of bed if unable to sleep within 20 minutes (20 minute rule) & spend quiet time in another room until noticing sleepiness signs again (to untrain a conditioned association of your bed with wakefulness).

7. Review/address sleep expectations (learn how heightened sleep expectations create anxiety, frustration and nervous system alertness). Paradoxical intention experiments targeting sleep expectations to reduce performance anxiety about sleep (by asking patients to do the most feared action: try to stay awake)

8. Worry and Rumination management skills.

'ALWAYS' ACTIONS

1. Acceptance & Values Review - nonjudgmental acceptance of our brain's oldest survival mechanisms: 1)fight or flee danger, and 2)get you to sleep. Building a quality of life around this.

THE MORNING AND DAYTIME ACTIONS
This may seem strange but when we start with resetting your sleep-wake cycle we will start with what you do in the morning. You may ask "Why aren't you focused on helping me get to sleep at night? That's where I'm having the problems!"

The reason for this is the nature of insomnia: unlike sleep deprivation where people have the ability to fall asleep but not the opportunity, in insomnia people have lots of opportunity to sleep but temporarily have lost the ability. Falling asleep, or sleep *onset*, is the one part that can't be guaranteed. As you've seen from the functions of anxiety in our evolution, if you're agitated enough, even with several sleep medications, your nervous system in fight-flight will resist sleep and try to override the sedatives to keep you scanning for threat. (In his last ten hours Michael Jackson was taking benzodiazepine doses every few hours after finishing dance rehearsal at 1am, but was still agitated and unable to initiate sleep). We can't guarantee your sleep onset but we *can* train your sleep backwards from your waking time using sunlight and homeostatic sleep pressure to compress your sleep.

So the essential habits and good sleep actions start with calibrating your circadian rhythm from your morning waking and rising.

1. SAME WAKING & RISING TIME EVERY DAY

Why? STRUCTURING YOUR DAY. Your brain works best being alert and awake in the daytime and resting and repairing in the night time. Daylight activity, exercise, and wakefulness, having early access to sunlight, and building purpose in our lives. Nighttime is for sleep, responsible for replenishing the brain and body, immunity, cell repair, and consolidating memory.

Melatonin sleep hormone is naturally produced in the pineal gland, from serotonin, as it gets dark. Core body temperature falls as melatonin production rises, and sleep readiness increases with these changes. As waking time nears in the morning your core body temperature rises, melatonin production turns down, and sleep urgency reduces. Then early morning sunlight entering your retina (even through closed eyelids) triggers waking via the SCN (suprachiasmatic nucleus) a wake-up clock in your brain, and triggers physical changes across your body (your adrenal activity, breathing rate, blood pressure, heart rate, metabolic rate, digestion, and more).

RESETTING YOUR CIRCADIAN CLOCK
Getting out of bed at the same time each day is more important in resetting your circadian clock than going to bed at the same time each night. There is no guarantee your sleep will start at the same time each night, even with a good bedtime routine habit. If you are agitated enough you will override even a strongly conditioned readiness to sleep at a certain time.

It's best to view this in terms of evolutionary strategy. This capacity to scan for and respond to threat is the oldest part of our brain. Every creature has the capacity to identify and respond to threat. Your survival depends on your brain being able to put aside sleep – at least for a period of time – while you deal with a threat. So, your brain can override your urge to sleep if there is a threat and you need to keep monitoring it. The threats might be different to 30,000 years ago, but the process is still as essential as ever, for survival. Because we can't ever guarantee sleep onset at a certain time, and in fact are likely to lose it if we try hard to fall asleep, we can only train from the waking time and morning sunlight to reset our circadian clock.

2. EARLY MORNING SUNLIGHT

Morning sunlight exposure resets your brain's sleep clock – your circadian rhythm - and your mood. Approximately 82% of our body's tissues have a circadian rhythm. As described earlier, early morning sunlight enters the retina and is transmitted to the SCN, or suprachiasmatic nucleus "wakeup clock" in the brain. This process triggers physical changes in the body that get you up and active. The SCN turns down melatonin sleep hormone production, while increasing blood pressure, metabolic rate, heart rate and breathing rate. Sunlight also improves serotonin neurotransmission, which is protective against depression. Just spending 30 minutes outside in morning sunlight will suppress melatonin, and ideally this is helped by not wearing tinted glasses or sunglasses. Hopefully there's no need to add that *no one* should look directly toward the sun in order to get sunlight exposure.

Finally, serotonin is used by the body in the manufacture of melatonin sleep hormone, which happens naturally as soon as darkness falls. So you start producing melatonin naturally after sunset. (Unless you go into a dark cinema for an after-lunch movie or close all your blinds for an afternoon nap).

What does affect normal melatonin production at night is use of electronic devices. If your device does not have a "red screen" download to filter out the blue wavelength of light (which your melanopsin photoreceptor is sensitive to) your brain will see this as akin to sunlight, and melatonin production will be suppressed to some degree.

3. RETRAIN A DELAYED CIRCADIAN SLEEP-WAKE SCHEDULE

If your natural waking time is more than 4 hours after dawn, set your alarm for your natural waking time and get at least 1 hour of sunlight or bright light exposure. Then on the next day and subsequent days set the alarm for 30 minutes earlier on each consecutive day (and get into the sunlight; don't return to sleep after the alarm sounds!) until goal waking & rising time is achieved.

Leon Lack at Flinders University in South Australia reinforces that our sleepiness and sleep "readiness" are strongly governed by our circadian clock via core body temperature. As you can see from the core temperature and sleep readiness graph featured earlier, the minimum core body temperature phase coincides with sleep. Higher core body temperature is associated with wakefulness.

A delayed sleep-wake schedule and delayed temperature rises and falls gets established with sleep onset insomnia. Morning bright light and dim light in evenings plus evening melatonin administration has been successful in "pulling back" core minimum body temperature and sleep readiness to earlier at night.

The important point is that the retraining of an earlier body temperature minimum needs to happen *gradually* as it becomes entrained over time to the later sleep onset. To put it simply, delayed waking equals delayed sleep onset. If you wake and rise at 11am it still takes approximately 14-16 waking hours to build up homeostatic sleep pressure, enough adenosine "sleep-inducer" and lowered core body temperature to get to sleep onset. If your natural waking time is delayed until 10-11am, then:

1) Your core temperature minimum is delayed until 8 AM to 9 AM, then
2) A "wakefulness zone" will occur from 10 PM to 2 AM, resulting in significant difficulty falling asleep until after 2 AM.

ADVANCED CIRCADIAN SLEEP-WAKE SCHEDULE: On the other hand too-early morning waking insomnia is associated with an advanced temperature rhythm and can be treated successfully with the delaying effect of evening bright light.

SLEEP MAINTENANCE INSOMNIA: (trouble staying asleep during the night) Disrupted sleep during the middle of the night (sleep maintenance insomnia) is actually linked not to a circadian rhythm timing problem, but to a generalized raised nighttime core body temperature. If you have a mixed sleep onset and sleep maintenance insomnia you may need to consider that you have chronically hypervigilant and "hyper-alert" central nervous system response to account for your chronically raised core body temperature. If this is the case and you are always in "fight-flight" you will need to work daily on relaxation strategies to teach your nervous system to quieten.

Here is an example of how your sleep diary would look with timed morning sunlight exposure if you have a delayed circadian sleep-wake cycle, and sleep onset problems:

So the process would start with your natural waking time of 12pm, then gradually marching the alarm clock and rising time back 30 minutes each day to allow your core body temperature to move back to an earlier minimum, until you get to an earlier waking and rising time (eg 7am) that works for you (which of course you would keep to, with consistent daily bright light exposure from 7am longterm :

To start: * Go to bed when sleepy _____ wake 30 min earlier (11:30)

                       * Go to bed when sleepy _____ wake 30 min earlier (11:00

                 * Go to bed when sleepy _____ wake up at same time (10:30)

             Etc.. (rise 30 minutes earlier every day with sunlight exposure).... Until:

To finish: * Go to bed when sleepy _____ wake 30 min earlier (7:00 a.m.)

See sleep diary example following:

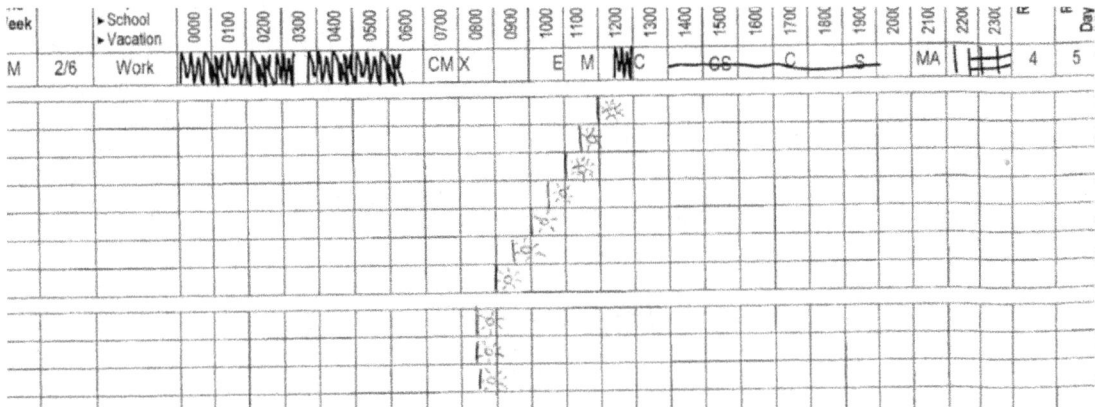

eek			0000	0100	0200	0300	0400	0500	0600	0700	0800	0900	1000	1100	1200	1300	1400	1500	1600	1700	1800	1900	2000	2100	2200	2300		Day
		►School ►Vacation																										
M	2/6	Work	⋀⋀⋀⋀⋀⋀⋀⋀	⋀⋀⋀⋀⋀⋀⋀	CM X			E	M	MC			CS		C		S		MA							4	5

HINTS:

Initial natural sleep time is about 2 AM to 12 pm and goal sleep time is between 11 PM and 7 AM. * means evening dim light and quiet, relaxing, nonstimulating activity before bedtime (no devices with blue wavelength light)

The sun symbol denotes morning bright light (sunlight or artificial light source).

4. AVOID DAYTIME NAPS, OR HAVE LESS THAN 30 MINUTE NAPS

Not napping during the day works to build up sleep "homeostatic" pressure over the day's waking hours. This is part of a coordinated response in insomnia CBT to relearn the bed=sleep association and maximize your chances of getting consolidated nighttime sleep. If you are suffering from insomnia currently it is best to keep to this strategy, even if you feel the urge to make up for lost sleep during the day. See the effect of daytime napping on sleep onset, below:

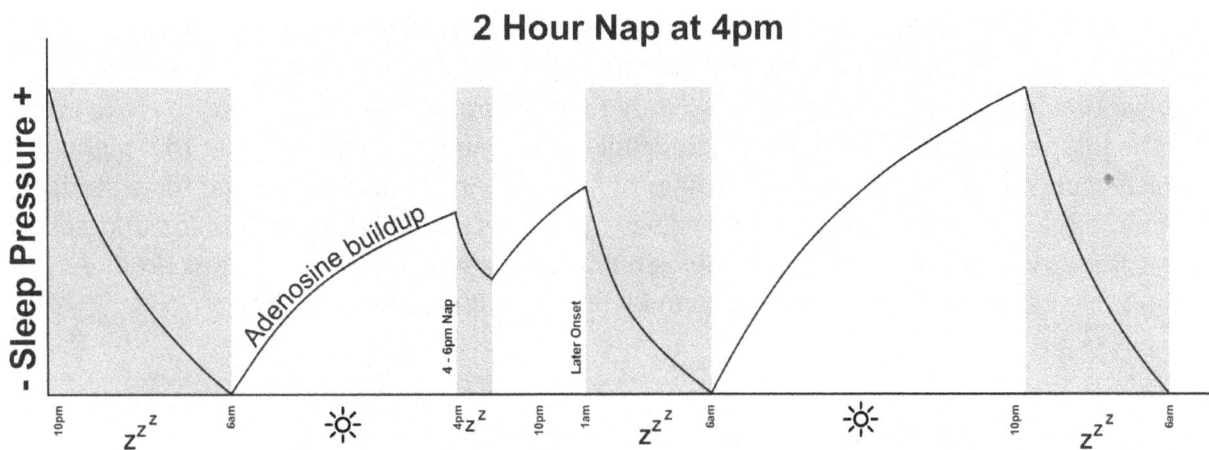

2 Hour Nap at 4pm

4.a) DAYTIME NAPPING AFFECTS SLEEP ONSET

Most people holding down study or jobs during business hours want a consolidated night-time sleep rather than late-onset or fragmented sleep. If you can avoid napping during the day, your brain will have much more adenosine "sleep-inducer", and pressure to sleep converging with darkness-generated melatonin (boosted by exposure to daytime sunlight), to get you sleepiness signals earlier in the night. This regular sleep-wake cycle (below) also benefits your mood.

Regular 8 hour sleep - wake pattern

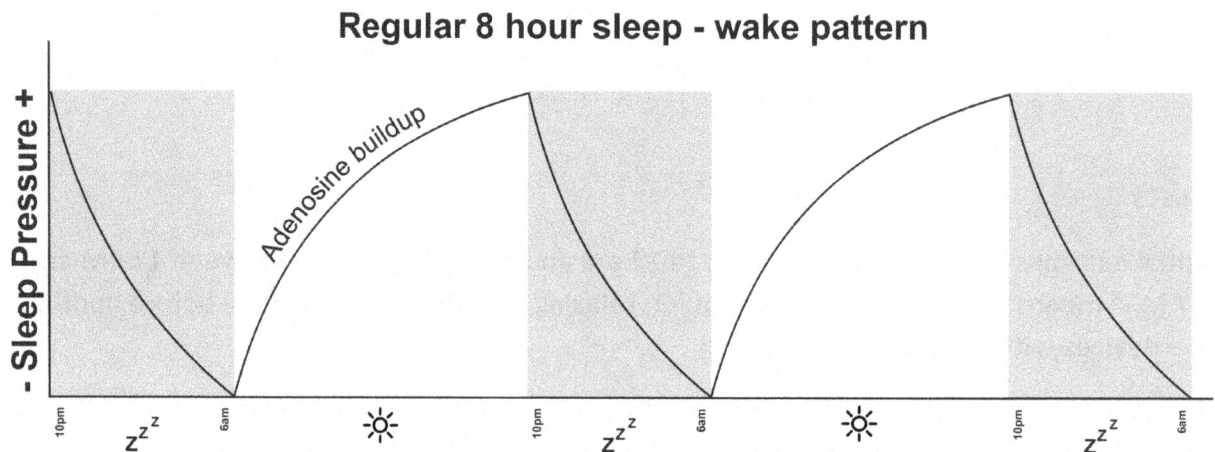

4.b) OBSTACLES TO AVOIDING NAPS: POST-LUNCH DROWSINESS AND L-TRYPTOPHAN

It's quite common to feel drowsy after lunch – our ultradian rhythm features a temporary drop in core body temperature in the early afternoon. This is accentuated if we eat tryptophan-rich protein foods (chicken, turkey, red meat, fish, eggs, dairy) for lunch.

L-tryptophan is an amino acid that your body converts into the B vitamin Niacin, which creates serotonin, the "sleep-related" neurotransmitter that the pineal gland uses to make melatonin sleep hormone.

Many people take the opportunity to nap after lunch, and a nap of about 20 minutes duration in the early afternoon will probably not weaken or dissipate your drive to sleep at night. However if you are currently suffering insomnia you may 1) want to "catch up" on sleep and have an urge to sleep for over an hour. (People with insomnia generally don't believe they've lost 20 minutes sleep, so they tend to nap for at least an hour to make up for the loss, and 2) then find yourself struggling with a much later sleep onset that night (which could condition more strongly the problem of laying in bed awake and frustrated). If insomnia is a problem it's better to stay away from naps and build more homeostatic sleep pressure during the day, so that you feel genuinely *drowsy* at bedtime, not just tired. As Colin Espie notes, naps don't cause insomnia, but they don't solve it either.

There are 2 qualifiers to add to this:

1) Most insomnia patients describe a day that is more "tired and wired", or tired and hyped-up, not *sleepy*. Many report that even if they wanted to and had opportunity to, they wouldn't be able to lay down and sleep during the day.
2) The exception is if there is objective drowsiness or sleepiness, and a history of microsleeps during the day, and especially if there is a question mark about excessive daytime sleepiness representing a specific sleep or breathing disorder, (eg a narcolepsy diagnosis or obstructive sleep apnoea diagnosis). Then it would be important to a) have an investigative sleep study and b) ensure adequate napping is scheduled during the day as required, especially if the person works with heavy machinery or in the heavy transport industry.

5. VIGOROUS EXERCISE EARLY IN THE DAY BUT ONLY A GENTLE STROLL AFTER 5PM

This section also relates to the night-time preparation actions. Energetic exercise during the day will not only help your mood but also your sleep quality – if you exercise early in the day. Unfortunately if you do vigorous exercise like jogging in the evening it may reduce your chances of getting to sleep because producing a large amount of adrenalin a few hours before bed will stimulate, not calm, your central nervous system. It may take 4-5 hours for your core temperature to cool down and nervous system to go back to baseline after vigorous exercise. So, jogging, dancing or brisk walking a few hours before bed may be too vigorous, but you can help along a relative drop in core temperature by doing very gentle exercise like a short stroll or low-stress yoga about 2 hours before bedtime. The degree of exercise strenuousness really matters for your sleep later in the evening.

NIGHT-TIME ACTIONS
GOAL: COOLING CORE BODY TEMPERATURE AND SLEEP

A drop in core body temperature of 1-2 degrees Celsius is needed to get to sleep and stay asleep. After a brief drop in core body temperature after lunch, which coincides with well-known post-lunch drowsiness, there is a mid or late afternoon rise, then a continuous drop in core body temperature until a minimum core temperature is reached 2-3 hours before morning waking.

AWAKE　　　　ASLEEP　　　AWAKE

Core Body Temperature

Sleepiness

Melatonin - Sleep Hormone

Minimum Core
Temp

| 8am | 10am | ☀ Midday | 2pm | 4pm | 6pm | 8pm | 10pm | 🌙 Midnight | 2am | 4am | 6am | 8am | 10am | ☀ Midday | 2pm |

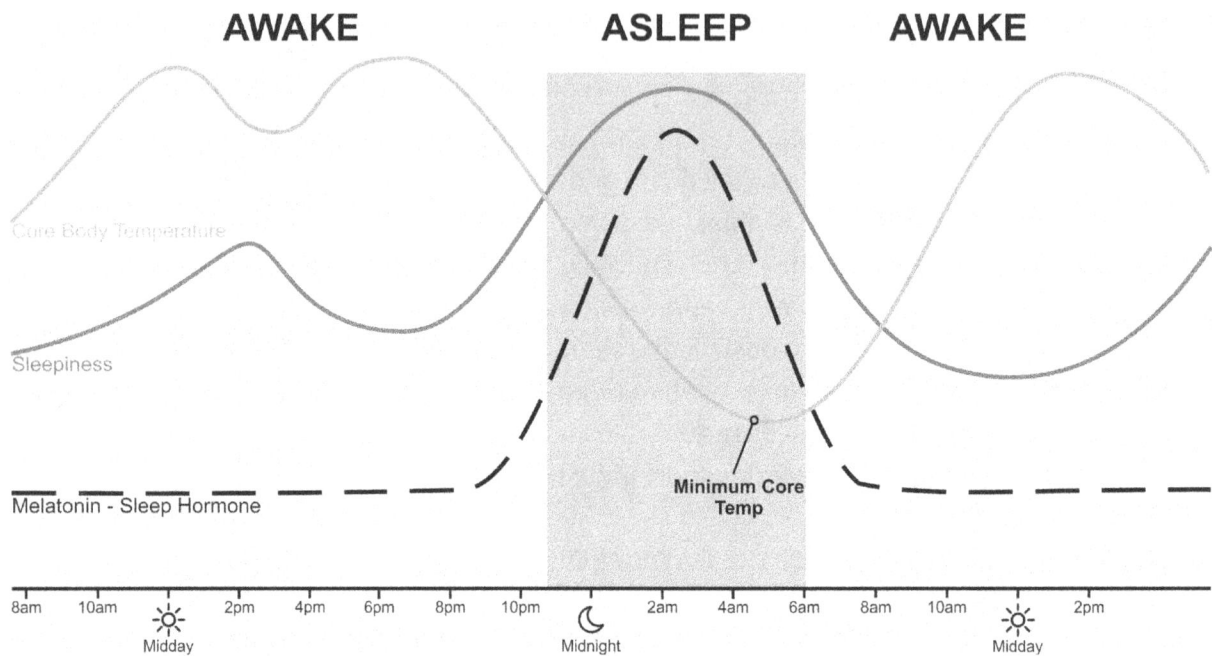

CORE BODY TEMPERATURE & SLEEPINESS:

There is also a wake maintenance zone in the hours before bed so just going to bed 2 hours early before your core temperature has been "entrained" to trigger sleep signals, will probably not get you sleep, and may create enough annoyance and bewilderment that your nervous system fires up again and the core temperature rise will then delay sleep more, even past your usual bedtime.

So, we need to work in with our naturally occurring and entrained body temperature drop as our brain and body ready us for sleep. We can also accentuate this drop in core temperature if we raise it by having a warm bath or shower about an hour before bedtime. The core temperature rises if we stay in the bath for around 30 minutes, then the relative drop in temperature in the next hour before bed will enhance our drowsiness.

1. **AVOID STIMULANT FOODS OR ACTIVITIES LATE IN THE DAY**

The reason to avoid stimulants (like nicotine or caffeine) before bed is stimulants tend to increase the heart rate, breathing rate and core body temperature. These physical changes will make it hard to get to sleep. The goal here is to learn about lifestyle and dietary insomnia triggers as part of basic sleep "hygiene", or core diet and lifestyle practices which aid your sleep regularity. It's also useful to understand the effects of stimulant intake and activities on your nervous system (sympathetic "fight-flight" responses) and how your thinking is affected by nervous system fight-flight hyperalertness.

CAFFEINE

Avoiding nervous system-stimulating caffeine in the late afternoon will reduce obstacles to sleepiness signals emerging that night. Avoiding coffee is not a guarantee of sleepiness, but will improve the chances of experiencing it after darkness falls. We usually talk about how long a substance's active effects on the brain are in terms of half-life. According to neuroscientist Matthew Walker the *quarter-life* of caffeine is 12 hours. This means if we drink a regular coffee at midday, then a quarter of that caffeine is still in the brain at midnight, a full 12 hours later, the effects ebbing away slowly. It's finally out of your system between 24 to 36 hours later. It's important to calculate how long that double shot espresso will be affecting your brain and nervous system as you try to stave off that post-lunch drowsiness.

RELAXATION SKILLS
As part of the wind down ritual to prepare for sleep, a nightly relaxation exercise for 15-20 minutes will also help to drop core body temperature. Going to bed with increased muscle tension as part of worry means more 1) thought processing, 2) attention monitoring, 3) emotion intensity, 4) adrenalin release, and general nervous system activity. This keeps us in semi-alert state as we scan for reasons to fight or flee. There is evidence that just having tense neck muscles keeps attached facet joints transmitting unnecessary proprioceptive information about the head's orientation to the brain through the night (but your brain doesn't need this continuous "orientation" information once your head is supported by your pillow). This is yet more biological feedback keeping your brain semi-alert through the night, and disrupting your sleep. So assume daily muscle relaxation and relaxed breathing exercises will be an important part of getting the nervous system to quiet down at the end of the day.

2. BUILD A SLEEP-FRIENDLY BED ENVIRONMENT TO HELP SLEEP ALONG

The bed should be a comfortable and uncluttered sleep environment to strengthen the bed-sleep connection. Any daytime or work-associated activities should be kept away from the bed. This includes laptops, phones, basically any electronic devices, both as blue wavelength light sources (physiological) and as associations with complex work planning and thinking activity (psychological association with wakefulness).

REDUCING NOISE
Reducing noise that might jolt you awake is a good part of a routine strengthening the bed-sleep connection. TV in particular has relative loudness increases during ad breaks, as well as brightness changes which can affect sleep onset. On the other hand, many people say they are lulled into sleep by the drone of a podcast or a late night radio announcer with a monotonous voice that is never raised. Meditation apps also help if people are unable to bat away intrusive thoughts when going to sleep. So the noise-reducing guideline is just that, not a rule to be kept to rigidly. The main goal is to start building a routine that your brain links to sleep, not wakefulness.

BEDROOM TEMPERATURE: SEASONS AFFECTING THE SLEEP ENVIRONMENT
In principle, a cooler rather than warmer bedroom (around 20-21 degrees Celsius) will assist the core body temperature drop into sleep. Many people with insomnia note they sleep better in winter than in summer, when the ambient temperature can make it hard to maintain a lowered body temperature.

Having said that, Seasonal Affective Disorder (SAD) is real, with objective sleep-worsening winter-time symptoms of low mood, low energy, poor concentration, constant tiredness, and inability to enjoy activities as before. It happens more as the days shorten in winter, so there are less sunlight hours. It affects people more the further they live from the equator. If people have a family history of depression in the cooler months, this may be more of a risk; a good working relationship with your medical practitioner will help to catch and treat this early with antidepressant medications that assist serotonin neurotransmission.

SAD Treatment involves:
Light Therapy (of 20-60 minutes each morning after waking) with light boxes providing about 20 times more light than regular indoor lighting, to help replace the sunlight being missed. Or SSRI (serotonin reuptake inhibitor) antidepressant medication to improve serotonin neurotransmitter activity (which will help the pineal gland in producing melatonin sleep hormone) and improve mood.

DARKNESS
As much as you can tolerate, your bedroom should be free from light. This is because your melanopsin photoreceptors are sensitive to light, especially blue-wavelength light from electronic devices. Even if you have a blue-light filter on your device you may find there is sufficient light to affect your melatonin production and delay sleep onset. Check your room for light-emitting devices like clocks. Clock-watching actually tends to raise anxiety about sleep. When people with insomnia see 1am on the clock their catastrophising bias usually makes them think they will never be able to fill the rest of the night with sleep, rather than how much extra time they have to enjoy sleep.

BEDROOM NOISE
Try to keep the bedroom free of any noise that can disturb your sleep, accepting that this will be more difficult in inner city areas. Noise is defined as any unwanted sounds that could affect you negatively psychologically and physically. A hyperacute hearing and nervous system response is the same in insomnia as it is in tinnitus. Irritant sounds take on threat meaning and set up a conditioned vigilant emotional response that leads to hypervigilant seeking out of more irritating sounds in the bed environment. Hence chapter 5 in this book is on managing over-attention to noise threats in insomnia.

3. TRAIN A BEDTIME RITUAL: A SERIES OF CONDITIONED ASSOCIATIONS BETWEEN YOUR BED AND SLEEPINESS

The overall longterm best-practice goal is: 1) to set up a reassuring bedtime routine that eases you toward 2) a non-negotiable 8-hour window of sleep OPPORTUNITY. Note this is an opportunity for sleep, not a guarantee of sleep; it just represents your valuing of sleep and creating enough space for it to go ahead.

REASONS FOR SETTING UP A BEDTIME RITUAL
The brain learns by building and strengthening associations (this will be explained in more detail in chapter 2). It rapidly builds connections – between toothbrushing and warm baths and imminent sleep. Or alternatively between the bed and wakefulness, so that the bed

and bedroom becomes a trigger, or cue, for alertness and complex problem-solving. Regularity is the key to building these connections: regularity in actions and habits will build you strengthened associations either toward sleep or away from it (for example, a habit of exposure to blue-wavelength light from electronic devices late at night affecting melatonin production and delaying sleep).

WHATEVER YOU PRACTISE, YOU GET GOOD AT
You know the phrase: whatever you practice, you get good at? That's what builds up associations and the neural pathways strengthening them. If you practice daily the same bedtime routine that results in sleep onset your brain comes to expect this and submit to it. Alternatively if you regularly practice lying awake in bed for hours, especially with associated dread and frustration, your brain comes to expect this also.

Normal Doidge's neuroplasticity research highlights how little cortex needs to be utilized once you have learned automatic behaviours and conditioned responses. For example, when you began to learn to drive, you needed to devote a large amount of concentrated attention and brain/cortical resources to learning to drive. After 20 years of regular driving you have reached maximum automaticity. It's a very efficient and economical process: your brain can free itself up for complex problem solving if all your driving actions are decided by a conditioned response template.

The only negative is that once you've trained into a conditioned association, you can't merely think your way out of it, even trying hard to problem solve. You have to act your way out of it, until another set of cues and responses becomes conditioned.
Behaviour change is difficult, especially as you need to keep repeating a new behavior if you want the behavior to become automatic, and get to a conditioned association. This is discussed in more detail in the sleep-safeguarding behaviours chapter.

A LIGHT CARBOHYDRATE SNACK AS PART OF A BEDTIME RITUAL

A light carbohydrate snack like rice or pasta can help induce sleep as part of a bedtime ritual. You'll recall that sleepiness is accentuated if we eat tryptophan-rich protein foods. And L-tryptophan is the amino acid that your body converts into the B vitamin Niacin, which creates serotonin, the neurotransmitter that the pineal gland uses to make melatonin sleep hormone. Well, carbohydrates react with your *stored* tryptophan to boost your serotonin neurotransmission, and enhance your pineal gland's melatonin production before bedtime. Also, psychologically many people report feeling comforted by a light snack before bed, fearing that gnawing hunger pangs may grab their attention and keep them awake.

4. GO TO BED WHEN SLEEPY TO ASSOCIATE BED WITH SLEEP

Going to bed when sleepy involves looking out for sleep "cues" or signals, like heavy head and eyelids, losing your place or missing lines if you're reading, or micro-sleeps where you notice blackness for a mere second then jerk awake in surprise. The hard part is just "letting" these signals come, if you've been worrying and no longer trust these signals.

Frantically seeking them will tend to work the other way, especially if your worry raises your core body temperature and creates hyperalertness for threat. Thankfully your brain is good at assessing night-by-night, how much homeostatic sleep pressure you've built, so you can resist it for only a finite period of time. The best thing is to focus on doing relaxation or an unstimulating activity without "laser-focus" attention, and your brain will generally take care of the sleep signals in the background.

5.HYPNOTIC SUBSTANCES (ALCOHOL, PRESCRIPTION SLEEP MEDICATIONS) & SEDATION

If you haven't started self-medicating for insomnia yet, try not to rely on hypnotic substances (alcohol, prescription sleep medications) before bedtime. Researcher Allison Harvey notes it's important to realise sedation is not the same as sleep. All hypnotic substances sedate the central nervous system to some degree, which mimics the downturn into sleep readiness and core body temperature drop that happens naturally. Hypnotics beckon you to the edge of sleep, but don't guarantee to tip you over into sleep. You may be surprised to find many people choose to go out and party after taking prescription hypnotics, not fall into sleep. If someone is agitated enough they can override the sedating effects and experience paradoxical wakefulness and central nervous system activation.

ALCOHOL:

How it feels: Alcohol initially sedates and relaxes, disinhibits, affects balance, coordination, memory and focus. As its effects wear off, it has the opposite effect: brain nerve stimulation and physical anxiety effects, the opposite of the sedation that was sought initially.

Effects on brain function: alcohol disrupts the normal balance existing between excitatory and inhibitory brain neurotransmitters, or biochemical messengers. Valenzuela (1997) explains how initially alcohol enhances inhibitory neurotransmitters (which depress the nervous system). But due to homeostasis the brain naturally attempts to fix the imbalance and restore equilibrium: by increasing excitatory neurotransmitters to compensate for alcohol's depressant effects. So when alcohol is taken away (withdrawal) the compensating excitatory effect keeps going and is no longer balanced by alcohol's inhibiting effects; the balance now tilts toward "hyper" (excess) excitation. This appears as anxiety, shaking, and even seizures in severe withdrawal. These withdrawal effects happen in both short-term and long-term alcohol use.

Specific effects on sleep: Alcohol increases cortisol release and raises core body temperature after the initial sedation, which affects ability to stay asleep through the night. Alcohol disrupts circadian rhythms, and because 82% of our body's tissues have a circadian rhythm, there are wide-ranging effects on the body: The liver's filtering function is compromised because of alcohol's disruption of the circadian clock's liver regulation. The gut is often seen as the second brain and is governed by circadian rhythms: alcohol influences leaky gut syndrome by weakening the lining of the gastrointestinal tract (allowing bacteria and toxins to leak through the gut into the bloodstream).

Alcohol suppresses melatonin sleep hormone (responsible for regulating sleep cycles) and REM (dream) sleep, causing difficulties with laying-down of new memory (REM sleep is important for both memory consolidation and emotion regulation). Recent research points to this increasing dementia risk over time, and alcohol-related brain damage is well known. Alcohol affects the sleep-wake cycle by reducing the responsiveness of the circadian drive to light cues that keep it on track.

Alcohol increases adenosine, a chemical marker of homeostatic sleep drive, which increases pressure to sleep at other times not dictated by your circadian rhythm, so disrupting your natural sleep-wake cycle.

Alcohol also increases the risk of accidental overdose because people often combine it with prescription sleep medications, not realizing the cumulative effect of slowing breathing. Depression is yet another result of disrupted circadian rhythms due to alcohol effects.

PRESCRIPTION HYPNOTIC/SLEEP MEDICATIONS

NEVER USED BEFORE BUT CONSIDERING:
If you have not yet used a prescription sleep medication give yourself 4-6 weeks to work on a psychological approach first before seeing your medical practitioner about pharmaceutical treatment. Remember key physician Colleges (The Royal Australian College of General Practitioners, the American College of Physicians) and professional bodies like The European Sleep Research Society all recommend Cognitive Behaviour Therapy as first-line treatment for insomnia, not hypnotic medication as first-line treatment. CBT and acceptance principles are the most effective treatment for insomnia and circadian sleep-wake problems. This Insomnia CBT program instills good sleep habits and flexible expectations which will help you regain trust and confidence in your sleep-regulation processes.

Four to six weeks will give you enough time to see the change in underlying conditioning and habit formation at work.

JUST BEGUN USING MEDICATIONS?
If you have just started using sleep medications first read the product information leaflet the pharmaceutical manufacturer has included in the pack (or download it and print out) and talk about it with your prescribing doctor.

Think of this as being just the start of your insomnia treatment exploration, not the end of the search. Plan firstly to be on the medication for 1-2 weeks and no more, just as the pharmaceutical company recommends. Even if your prescribing doctor is easygoing about "just use it when you need it". Because the dopamine reward pathway is involved and because people are so relieved with the sedation and non-recall of waking, it very quickly turns into a nightly must-have. This then leads into the issue of desensitization, tolerance to the medication, and learned helplessness as a result of medication tolerance.

If dependent on sleep medications, establish with your doctor a tapering regime to reduce alongside this CBT program. The goal is to understand why we attribute sleep to substances, and learn good sleep habits and ways to quiet the nervous system instead of depending on sedative and hypnotic medications to get to sleep.

6. STIMULUS CONTROL THERAPY: GET OUT OF BED IF UNABLE TO SLEEP IN 20 MINUTES: UNTRAINING A CONDITIONED ASSOCIATION BETWEEN BED AND WAKEFULNESS

The goals in insomnia CBT are to regulate your sleep/wake cycle and to change behavior habits and thinking biases about sleep. The plan is ultimately to reassociate bed with sleep, instead of the frustration and anxiety that are associated with continually laying awake in bed over time.

THE PROCEDURE:
The procedure with the traditional "20 minute rule" is to recognize when you have been unable to sleep for around 20 minutes and then get yourself out of bed and spend quiet time in another room until you notice sleepiness signs again. The goal is to untrain a conditioned association of your bed with wakefulness. Most people can't see the point in doing this because they don't really understand the underlying associative learning (that by staying in bed you are gradually and unconsciously "pairing" your bed with frustrated wakefulness and other strong emotions). Also they just don't want to, especially in winter, with hopeful thoughts like "maybe even resting in bed is as good" keeping them in bed.

So, just to recap on associative learning, yes, it's really important to do the 20 minute rule to ultimately overcome a conditioned association of your bed with waking, worrying and threat-monitoring. You can't think your way out of a conditioned association precisely because making habits automatic is exactly what your brain is good at doing. Once you've paired two previously unrelated things until they're habitual, your brain literally ignores the association, to get on with other pressing higher-order thinking activities, like worry and rumination and problem-solving not sleeping.

HOW TO GO ABOUT IT?
To reassociate the bed itself with sleep, and overturn a conditioned association of the bed with worry-infused waking (a process called sleep consolidation) start by imagining sleep as a piano accordion, which you stretch and squeeze to get musical notes. In sleep consolidation, we are squeezing out the unwanted waking and worrying periods that strengthen the bed-awake association.

As mentioned, the usual trigger for deciding to get out of bed is the 15 or 20 minute rule. You get out of bed if you've been awake for 15-20 minutes. Or, put another way, if you can't get back to sleep within 15-20 minutes you get up and go to another room where you do something unstimulating but relaxing (like meditation, muscle relaxation, or breathing mindfulness) until you feel sleepy again. You then take this sleepy feeling back to your bedroom, and give yourself another chance to sleep. Without trying or any sort of mental effort.

The problem is, what if you can't tell if it has been 15-20 minutes? What if it feels like at least half an hour but you have been told your subjective impression doesn't match up with the actual time that's passed. (Many people find out in a sleep study that they have not been awake as long as they believe they have been). This is where the common "Sleep State Misperception" comes in. Many people misperceive their waking periods as being much longer than they actually are, just because they have a strong belief they have been awake for a long time (for example believing 11 minutes awake duration on polysomnography was over 1 hour awake).

Many people have sleep-state misperception, thinking they are awake for much longer than they really are. A lot of focused thinking and awareness of the environment goes on during the light sleep stages 1 and 2. If you already 1) overvalue sleep, and 2) have a bias for assuming your sleep is poor or inadequate, then you will already have a confirmatory and selective attentional bias for listening out for evidence of this. That means hearing things in your environment that other people would ignore and memorizing them as evidence that your theory of poor sleep is correct. This is why a bias is called selective (focusing mainly on the data that supports your theory) and confirmatory (settling your attention on information that confirms your theory's right). We will explore this in more detail in the chapter on belief and expectation barriers to change, and try to provide reassuring information to aid belief change.

Understandably it's a difficult goal deciding to get out of bed so that the bed is not paired with wakefulness. Getting out of bed is seen as aversive, so there's no clear immediate reward or positive reinforcement we can easily make a habit with. You'll need to investigate your reasons, your longer term "whys" for getting out of bed to work on conditioning processes. This is where the motivational work in the Values chapter can help.

RESTRICTING TIME IN BED TO APPROXIMATE NUMBER OF HOURS SLEPT
TO CONSOLIDATE SLEEP:
This is the alternative to the 15 minute rule if you suffer from Sleep State Misperception. It works rapidly to build homeostatic sleep pressure to compress your sleep into a consolidated block, with mild sleep deprivation. Let's say you believe you only sleep 6 hours a night, then the starting sleep window from lights out to final rising time would be restricted to 6 hours. Ongoing alterations to this sleep window are based on your sleep efficiency (the percentage of time spent in bed that you've actually slept) until your brain's natural sleep baseline emerges.
Example:

Time actually slept: **6** hours vs **9** hours spent in bed = **3** hours awake & frustrated in bed
_____6hr sleep
_____**3hr awake** 9hr total time in bed

We need to squeeze out this 3 hours wakefulness and frustration per night, as it strengthens a conditioned association pairing your bed with being awake & frustrated. The plan is to take that wakefulness and frustration to the sofa in another room, so that your sofa is associated with wakefulness and strong emotion and your bed is only associated with sleep. That means 3 hours extra on your lounge, either before or after your consolidated 6 hour sleep opportunity.

If you have Sleep State Misperception and you aren't sure but you think you're awake, the plan is to assume you're awake and take the doubt, yearning, and frustration out to the sofa anyway.

You may be thinking "what to do out on the sofa for 3 hours?" More than ever, relaxation skills, meditation apps, quiet reading, are necessary to keep your motivation up during this process. Expect loss of motivation – it's inevitable with restricting time in bed, and it often leads to dropout mainly because people don't see how sunlight and homeostatic pressure can work together to compress and train the sleep window. On the plus side, it doesn't take too many days to work if you're committing to it, as your brain is faithfully calibrating and calculating if sleep deprivation needs correcting in the background. The trick is to put your faith in your homeostatic drive and start this on your week off work or study.

7. REVIEW/ADDRESS SLEEP EXPECTATIONS

Heightened expectations about sleep create anxiety, frustration & cortical and nervous system hyperalertness. Reviewing and addressing unrealistic sleep expectations helps us let go of such fears as getting inadequate sleep will make us useless the next day. Addressing expectations works to combat another irony of insomnia that Charles Morin highlighted: that people who have difficulties with sleep tend to expect more out of it than people who don't (because of both overvaluing sleep and overestimating cost and likelihood of the worst happening).

People with insomnia tend to think that one night of poor sleep leads to health problems or has a crushing impact the next day and so must be avoided at all cost. This sets up a mental pressure-cooker that leaves them fretting that every second they are awake in the middle of the night is making catastrophe more likely. In the inverted logic of insomnia, sleep is extremely important to someone with insomnia. And therefore, the person with insomnia can't get sleep.

PARADOXICAL INTENTION EXPERIMENTS:

These experiments target expectations to reduce performance anxiety about sleep by asking patients to do their most feared action: *try to stay awake* (and keeping eyes open- but avoiding devices). These are explored further in the behaviour experiments chapter.

8. WORRY AND RUMINATION MANAGEMENT SKILLS

Because Worry and Rumination are such an intrinsic part of insomnia it will be important to train in worry and rumination management skills. The second half of Chapter 8 is on worry and rumination and follows on from the Beliefs and Expectations thought recording and evidence-gathering skills.

'ALWAYS' ACTIONS

1.ACCEPTANCE AND VALUES REVIEW-

This is about allowing nonjudgmental acceptance of our brain's oldest survival mechanisms: 1) fight or flee danger, and 2)get us to sleep. The goal is building a quality of life around these realities, working with our brain and not against it. Please see the Values review chapter later in this book.

CHAPTER 7   UNDERSTANDING SLEEP BELIEFS AND EXPECTATIONS

This section of the book is about your beliefs and expectations about sleep, the attributions driving threat monitoring and those backfiring sleep safety-seeking actions. We explore sleep expectations barriers to trying insomnia solutions or testing out unhelpful insomnia beliefs.

PERCEPTIONS LINK TO FEELINGS AND ACTIONS

You'll recall in chapter 2 we talked of how, when we are sleepless, THOUGHTS lead to EMOTIONS lead to ATTENTION lead to SAFETY-SEEKING ACTIONS, in a sleep "hypervigilance" (hyperalertness) loop:

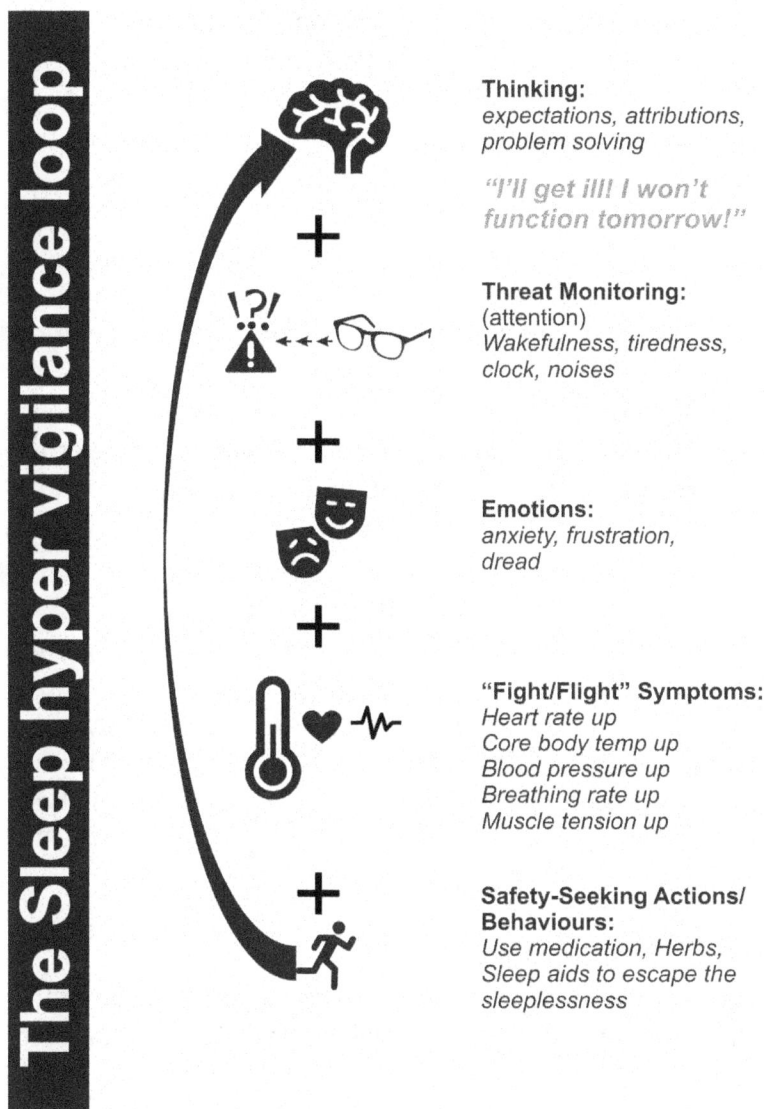

The Sleep hyper vigilance loop

Thinking:
expectations, attributions, problem solving

"I'll get ill! I won't function tomorrow!"

Threat Monitoring:
(attention)
Wakefulness, tiredness, clock, noises

Emotions:
anxiety, frustration, dread

"Fight/Flight" Symptoms:
Heart rate up
Core body temp up
Blood pressure up
Breathing rate up
Muscle tension up

Safety-Seeking Actions/ Behaviours:
Use medication, Herbs, Sleep aids to escape the sleeplessness

Many people believe that external events, situations or people are responsible for determining the feelings/emotions they experience. But we come to this conclusion without asking ourselves if we're assuming incorrectly. What actually makes us feel and respond in a certain way is how we *perceive* the person's actions or the situation.

AUTOMATIC HABITS OF THINKING

We're not always aware of our attributions of causation or responsibility; often it happens so rapidly and automatically that we don't catch up the role of our thoughts and feelings about someone or something. We've become so practised at thinking along certain lines that we've accepted this perspective as normal. It's a bit like being on automatic pilot when we drive a car, and let automatic, habitual thoughts through unchallenged. Just like driving, when our thinking and attention are so habitual after following the same line longterm, we're just not aware or conscious of them.

COGNITIVE THERAPY AND EVIDENCE BASE

As described earlier, there is neuroplasticity research and habit formation research that support this. We've looked at how the major sleep and medical organisations have released guidelines recommending cognitive behaviour therapy as the first-line treatment for insomnia. These recommendations have been reached after reviews of hundreds of insomnia research studies, pulled together in what's called a "meta-analysis". When organisations say cognitive and behaviour therapy is "evidence-based" they're referring to these meta-analytic reviews of hundreds of studies featuring thousands of treatment subjects.

Many people think cognitive therapy is just about replacing a negative thought with a positive thought. But it's definitely not simply trying to think positive thoughts as a solution to sleep problems. This is especially the case with sleep because you can't put a positive spin on real sleep deprivation – it not only feels terrible; there are real negative consequences to insomnia including deteriorating into depression over time. We need to take insomnia seriously because of the reciprocal relationship between insomnia and mental health problems.

COGNITIVE THERAPY: WEIGHING THE EVIDENCE AND UNCOVERING BIASES

Cognitive therapy focuses on the value of weighing the evidence for and against fears, and considering as many different angles on a problem as possible. Often we have spent so long in certain habits of thinking that we have formed errors and biases, or biased thinking and attention about a certain issue. Viewing an insomnia problem from different perspectives – brainstorming on negative, positive and neutral aspects or outcomes of insomnia – will help us uncover our biases or "blind spots" and increase our chances of finding creative solutions.

FAULTY AND UNHELPFUL THINKING HABITS IN INSOMNIA

Here are a few of the types of habitual thinking errors and biases that understandably start developing once we've started conditioning insomnia's worry and hypervigilance to our bed environment:

- Misconceptions, misattributions re causes of insomnia ("I have lost the ability to sleep"; "my sleep mechanism is defective/broken"; "I have a biochemical imbalance")

- Misattributions and catastrophic beliefs re insomnia consequences (all daytime impairments and health impacts are caused by poor sleep: "I can't concentrate at all because I slept so badly!" "This poor sleep will get me fired!"; "poor sleep is making me sick")

- Unrealistic sleep expectations ("I should have 8 hours sleep every night")

- Beliefs about diminished control over & predictability of sleep ("I will never sleep properly again", "I've got no control over my sleep– now I'll have to stay on medications the rest of my life")

- Misconceptions about strategies to promote sleep ("I'll get more sleep if I just spend more time in bed"; "the medication will take care of it for me")

- Thinking styles: Black & white ("My sleep is just bad from start to finish") selective attention ("I only got 2 hours sleep last night", and emotional reasoning "if it feels like I'm not sleeping, then I'm not sleeping!")

- Rigid rules about sleep:
    - Sleep should be controllable through sleep effort, More effort should bring more sleep
    - Poor sleep = expect poor daytime energy, poor functioning, poor focus, poor memory
    - Good sleep =expect good daytime energy, good functioning, good focus, good memory
    - "quantity = quality"; "8 hrs = mandatory"; 1hr extra sleep in am = "critical" for daytime functioning

INTERNAL VS EXTERNAL LOCUS OF CONTROL

When people have a strong belief that they have agency and some control over their sleep and can influence their sleep quality, this is called an internal locus of control. On the other hand, someone with an external locus of control might believe they have little or no control over their sleep neurochemistry and that an external agent or medication will be needed to get them more or better sleep.

People with an internal locus of control will be responsive to the idea that you can change your sleep by changing your habits or learning CNS-calming breathing or relaxation skills.

People with an external locus of control will be more likely to trust an external sleep aid (like alcohol or medications) to influence their neurochemistry and sedate their nervous system.

Which statement more closely resembles the way you feel about sleep:

I believe insomnia results from a chemical imbalance and sleep medication will restore balance:

Strongly agree..Strongly disagree

Or

I believe I can learn skills and change habits to get a better sleep pattern:

Strongly agree..Strongly disagree

Neither one is good or bad, it's just helpful to get an insight into our basic beliefs and thinking styles. Then we'll know what we're working with and why some of the strategies in this workbook might be more of a struggle.

ATTRIBUTIONS OF CAUSATION

Attributions are how an insomnia sufferer interprets a night's poor sleep. Because we generally all try to understand and problem-solve poor sleep, we're trying to find something to attribute it to. Something internal or something external. We might attribute our poor sleep to the coffee we drank at 2pm if we know something about the half-life or active effects of caffeine on our brain chemistry. We might then attribute our yawning mid-morning to the poor sleep we had last night. If we're feeling trapped in a stressful job we might attribute our poor sleep to the job demands.

Which statement more closely resembles your attributions of poor sleep:
When I sleep badly I think it's because of something I must have done during the day or before bed:
Strongly agree..Strongly disagree
Or
My sleep's always bad because my brain chemistry is out of balance:
Strongly agree..Strongly disagree

You may have your own theories or attributions about your good and bad sleep. Write down your thoughts on these:
When I sleep well I believe it's generally because: ....
When I sleep badly I believe it's generally because:...

If we have an internal locus of control we might then look for something within our control as we attribute sleeplessness, like exercising late or working too late and not having enough wind-down time. Something that we can work on the next day to bring about a better sleep. If we have an external locus of control we might prioritise getting to the pharmacy to fill a medication script rather than book into a regular meditation class to help sleep.

EXPECTATIONS RISE WITH MORE BEDTIME ROUTINES AND SLEEP AIDS

This is part of the paradox of insomnia. As more sleep aids are tried and more "sleep-inducing" routines are added in, the more expectations of success arise. And unfortunately the more monitoring for effectiveness increases. A 45 minute bedtime routine kept to rigidly can reflect a lot of expectation of sleep success. This also reflects and confirms a lot of doubt, uncertainty and performance anxiety about sleep.

EXPECTATION AND BIAS

Thinking and attention bias is informed by and also confirms insomnia sleep expectations. The strong belief "I won't get good sleep" or "my sleep is fragile" will lead us to selective monitor wakefulness and tiredness symptoms and search for more and more sleep aids and routines to try to "guarantee" sleep. This means we will be putting more of our attention on to whether our new routines and sleep aids are doing what they're supposed to do (make sleep happen). This makes us expect more from sleep than unworried sleepers do. Unfortunately, with all this thought and attention focused on preventing the threat of not sleeping, not sleeping becomes more likely: a self-fulfilling prophecy. Our central nervous system is on high alert looking for evidence that the new routine or sleep aid is working. Our frontal lobe is already sizing up reality against our sleep expectations, and readying itself to problem-solve if things aren't working out.

This goes back to accepting our brain's sleep self-regulation and whatever baseline sleep it gives us. The Balance here will be to value, not overvalue sleep. If we overvalue sleep, we then demand more of it and want guarantees it will not only happen, but happen "well".

BARRIERS TO TRYING GOOD SLEEP HABITS
It's quite understandable that the core "Good Sleep' Habits in the last chapter will not look very appealing if you have insomnia. After all, many of the sleep safeguarding or sleep safety-seeking actions in insomnia go against these.
Let's look back at the core habits and try to capture what will be difficult about doing them.

LetSleepHappen Sleep Program Core Good habits and learning objectives:
Again, these are the essential actions needed to regulate your sleep-wake cycle and pave the way to (with the learning objectives alongside each). This time, write down why you think you won't be able to do these actions: it's okay to admit you can't see yourself doing any of them. At least you'll know what levels of fear or belief strength you have about sleep.

- Same waking and rising time daily (to align with the sun rising, & to reset sleep wake schedule in accord with the body's internal circadian rhythms)
- I don't believe this would work for me because:…………………………………………………

  ………

- Early morning sunlight (to turn off melatonin sleep hormone production and reset your circadian rhythm, governed by light and darkness).
- I don't believe this would work for me because:…………………………………………………

  ………

- No naps during the daytime if you have current insomnia, to build up homeostatic pressure over the day's waking hours (a 20-30 min nap is okay if no insomnia)
- I don't believe this would work for me because:…………………………………………………

  ………

- Exercise during day but no later than 5pm (for muscle relaxation, and to accentuate the body's natural parasympathetic/calming nervous system response before bed)
- I don't believe this would work for me because:…………………………………………………

  ………

- Follow a regular bedtime wind-down routine (using associative learning principles, to associate your bed with sleep & strengthen this paired association over time)
- I don't believe this would work for me because:…………………………………………………

  ………

- Go to bed only when sleepy (to increase your chances of bed being associated with sleep, and reduce your chances of bed being associated with wakefulness)

- I don't believe this would work for me because:…………………………………………………
  ………

- Get out of bed if unable to sleep within 20 minutes (20 minute rule) and spend quiet time in another room until noticing sleepiness signs again (to untrain a conditioned association of your bed with wakefulness)
- I don't believe this would work for me because:…………………………………………………
  ………

- If your natural waking time is more than 4 hours after dawn, set alarm for natural waking time & get exposure to bright light. Then set alarm for 30 minutes earlier on each subsequent day (and get up immediately after your alarm sounds) until goal waking & rising time is achieved, and early morning sunlight exposure occurs. (to overturn a delayed circadian sleep-wake disorder)
- I don't believe this would work for me because:…………………………………………………
  ………

- No stimulants (nicotine, caffeine) or stimulant activity before bed (to understand lifestyle and dietary triggers to insomnia, as part of basic sleep "hygiene", or practices to help sleep regularity. Also understanding your sympathetic ('ON") vs parasympathetic ("OFF") nervous system responses)
- I don't believe this would work for me because:…………………………………………………
  ………

- Dark or near-darkness, cooler ambient temperature, reduced noise in sleep environment (to calm CNS and condition sleepiness to bedtime ritual/bed environ)
- I don't believe this would work for me because:…………………………………………………
  ………

- Catch/address/Modify sleep expectations (to learn how high expectations about sleep create anxiety, frustration & more hypervigilance)
- I don't believe this would work for me because:…………………………………………………
  ………

- Long term, not relying on hypnotic substances (alcohol, prescription sleep medications) before bed. DO NOT STOP ALCOHOL OR SLEEPING PILLS SUDDENLY IF YOU HAVE BEEN USING THEM DAILY FOR OVER 6 MONTHS. Consult your medical practitioner first if you wish to reduce any hypnotic substance or medication. If you rely on sleep medications daily you and your doctor can consult on a tapering regime to reduce alongside this CBT program (goal is to understand attributing sleep to substances, and preparedness to learn sleep habits & calm CNS on own vs depend on sedative & hypnotic medications to get to sleep). There is a detailed chapter on how to go about this in the second half of this book.

- I don't believe this would work for me because:………………………………………………………
……

Please move straight on to the next chapter which is on *testing* sleep beliefs and expectations which are barriers to getting out of insomnia.

CHAPTER 8   TESTING INSOMNIA BELIEFS & EXPECTATIONS

Let's revisit the beliefs and expectations behind the barriers to change, and this time also try to answer the fears that keep people doing them. We'll look at reassuring information to promote acceptance of our brain's sleep regulation, and core sleep habit change.

Understandably, if it isn't reassuring enough, sleepless people won't get out of bed to reassociate their bed with sleep. If it isn't reassuring enough, insomnia sufferers attributing sleep success to sleep medications just won't have the confidence to try to come off them. You're not alone if this is your situation; researchers across the world are highlighting the clear difficulty in stopping sleep medications becoming a longterm dependence, which shows just how readily people attribute sleep control and success to the medications.

The tool we'll use for this is a thought record, because this is how we gather and weigh real evidence for and against our fears, and how we uncover our own thinking biases. We all do this, skewing incoming information and selectively perceiving ourselves and the world around us. Because we all have theories about the world and we're all interpreting what happens to us and inside us in a way that confirms our theories. Hence our unexamined biases are selective and confirmatory. The job of the thought record is to test this out (below).

My negative (fearful, frustrated) thoughts about sleep	How these thoughts make me feel	Evidence For fearful thought ie cost **will be severe** if poor sleep	Evidence against fearful thought ie cost **will not be severe** if poor sleep	Balanced, alternative thought	How I feel now
Example: If my sleep doesn't get better I'll get sacked- I just can't focus	frustrated 80% -about poor sleep scared 90% - about my job	Boss noticed a mistake on my report. I wasn't focused when I wrote it because of my tiredness.	He praised the report. I'm focusing on one mistake and blaming it on my sleep. I've made mistakes after a good night's sleep too.	My focus is OK if I'm interested, & not under time pressure; it's not just about sleep	10% scared re job
Your example:					
The thoughts/images on my mind	Emotion/ feeling 0-100% intensity	Past facts, events support big/severe cost eg sleep rule: poor sleep=poor energy, focus, functioning good sleep=good energy, focus, memory, functioning	Past facts/events show cost will not be big/severe, as expected. Some experiences not supporting rule; facts show I overestimate danger	Balanced view that allows for both evidence for & against fearful thought	Emotion intensity 0-100% after testing thought

The first column is where we record our frustrated or anxious thoughts about sleep or daytime tiredness. The second column is where we record how we feel having those thoughts. Then the third column is where we record evidence *for* a severe cost or impact on us if we get poor sleep. The fourth column is where we counter that evidence, this time collecting evidence *against* a severe impact or cost if we get poor sleep.

The last two columns are where we incorporate both the likelihood of severe impact *and* likelihood of coping with it, using whatever past and present evidence we have collected. This process of writing itself will allow us to uncover biases and assumptions we haven't questioned before. And the last column is where we record how we feel after completing this investigation. The bottom row of the record has prompts to help us gather evidence from our past about rules

CATCHING THINKING AND ATTENTION BIAS IS HARD WORK

Overcoming a thinking bias is hard, mainly because we've been filtering incoming information for so long in habitual ways we just don't know we're doing it. The whole process is unquestioning. Thinking and attention biases are selective and confirmatory by their nature; we tend to selectively collect or allow evidence that supports what we already believe, while ignoring other important evidence that could lead to a very different interpretation. And we need to catch bias in order to question it.

When we have insomnia we selectively find evidence for the beliefs 1) bad sleep and bad daytime consequences will be very likely to happen to me, and 2) will severely cost/impact me and I won't be able to cope. Let's just assume thoughts like this are on our minds if we ticked all the insomnia diagnosis boxes in chapter 1 (we may be more or less aware of them under stress). Understandably these would be good reasons people would not want to, for example, get out of bed to unlearn a conditioned association of bed and wakeful frustration or fear. The hope is that with a) understanding about conditioning and habit formation, b) knowing what your sleep does in the background to help you, and c) allowing that there are ways to think differently about sleep, you can feel confident to persevere with CBT strategies.

SEARCHING TO CONFIRM BIASED BELIEFS ABOUT POOR SLEEP

When we have sleep difficulties we usually start with the belief that we don't sleep more than a short number of hours per night, and look for data confirming that this is true. For example our attention will be more focused on tiredness and low energy signs in the daytime, as evidence we only slept a short time. We will selectively recall clock times very well, as evidence we were awake much of the night. At the same time we wouldn't focus attention on when we lost track of time during the night, or the bits that didn't make sense and were probably dreams or light sleep stages.

UNCOVERING BIAS & WEIGHING EVIDENCE FOR AND AGAINST MY FEARS

Some of the best questions to help us uncover an unconsciously operating bias are:

- "Is there another way to look at this?"
- "What real facts support my fears, that are not just based on my feelings?"
- "Are there any, even small, experiences, which contradict my expectations and surprise me?"

EXCEPTIONS TO RIGID RULES: CATCH THE SURPRISES!

- Rigid rules raise threat, raise sleep performance anxiety and prompt safety behaviours that backfire.

- Instead try raise curiosity re "surprises" (times when we functioned poorly despite good sleep, and vice versa. Times when we notice quantity is not equal to quality, and sleeping more means feeling worse upon waking (often found in a regular sleep diary).

- Test the need for optimal alertness in the daytime cycle of sleep threat (about "getting it wrong"? what's the worst outcome? What was the worst that happened in the past? Just how likely is the worst outcome?).

Any evidence that is an exception to the rules "Good Sleep = Good Energy/functioning", or "Poor Sleep = Poor Functioning/Energy" should be noted and put in the thought record. We can overcome a bias if we open out our attention to allow surprises like this:
"It's true I feel tired but I still manage to get things done ok at work. In fact, some of my best functioning happens after a "bad" night because I'm more likely to focus hard on getting my work out of the way, and less likely to chat with colleagues!"
And :
"I've made mistakes at work on days where I've had a good night's sleep prior".
And:
Reassuring thoughts which challenge a bias: There are actually some things (like create energy) I can do to manage my tiredness feelings during the day, so I'm not helpless.

Let's look at Sleep State Misperception, (or paradoxical insomnia, because people believe they have not been sleeping even when objective data shows they are sleeping). Sleep state misperception is not necessarily separate from insomnia. In fact, as Allison Harvey notes, people start off with a perception that their sleep is poor that conditions worry and wakefulness in bed to such an extent that the hypervigilance creates objectively disrupted sleep. An important piece of evidence, however, is a key review of Chambers & Keller (1993) which found only a 35 minute average difference between insomnia sufferers and untroubled sleepers.

IS THERE A BIAS IN SLEEP STATE MISPERCEPTION?

It is very common for humans to misjudge 1)how long it takes us to fall asleep, 2)the duration of our sleep, & 3)quality of sleep. Because there is no awareness or memory for the moment we fall asleep (but a strong awareness of the time we wake during the night) we tend to skew the data and estimate we were awake for much longer than we actually were. We know this because it is very common for people's perceptions of sleep timing and duration to not match up with objective polysomnography data from their sleep lab study. Time awake during the night is also seen to pass more slowly because there is an absence of anything to distract us. And this is something we get stuck worrying about, during both night and day. The only times recalled are overtly negative emotionally-meaningful awake periods.

My negative (fearful, frustrated) thoughts about sleep	How these thoughts make me feel	Evidence For fearful thought ie cost **will be big** if poor sleep	Evidence against fearful thought ie cost **will not be big** if poor sleep	Balanced, alternative thought	How I feel now
I'm just not sleeping; I don't know how the sleep study didn't find that!	frustrated 80% and bewildered 90% about discrepancy between self-report and sleep data	It didn't feel like I slept more than an hour. If I feel so tired I must have slept badly!	The sleep study data says I was sleeping. My fitbit says I sleep well. I do feel tired from worrying. On days off work I don't worry and I don't feel tired, even if I sleep less.	*I can't judge the time that I'm asleep because that time feels like an absence- I only recall the waking time . Worry exhausts me more than fragmented sleep*	Frustrat'n 10%; bewilderd 0%
The thoughts/images on my mind	Emotion/feeling 0-100% intensity	Past facts, events support big/severe cost eg sleep rule: poor sleep=poor energy, focus, functioning	Past facts/events show cost will not be big/severe, as expected, so don't support rule; facts show I overestimate danger	Balanced view that allows for both evidence for & against fearful thought	Emotion intensity 0-100% after testing thought

Here is some specific evidence of selective & confirmatory bias about nighttime wakefulness:

1. During a night in a sleep lab, people with insomnia often complain it took more than an hour to fall asleep when the polysomnography data shows sleep onset within 10 minutes. Estimated duration is also skewed, with many perceiving they didn't sleep at all despite hours of video and brain wave evidence to the contrary.

2. We can't easily judge the time that we are asleep because **that time feels like an absence**, a break from the demands of thought and awareness. The times that we do remember are those that we wish we couldn't: staring at the clock in the middle of the night, turning the pillow over desperately hoping that the other side is cooler, kicking the covers off or pulling them up close.

3.Even if awake time is only 3 minutes, because of our fears the experiences can become exaggerated in our minds and overshadow the hours that we were sleeping peacefully, simply because we *remember them too well*. And we recall them selectively because they confirm our existing hypothesis about our sleep being poor. Charles Morin's research also found evidence of patients with insomnia recalling stage 1 & 2 sleep too well.

The special challenges in gathering evidence around Sleep State Misperception are:

- There are usually no clearcut wakefulness periods, either on polysomnography data or in sufferers' self-report; insomnia clients will feel they have been dozing all night or semi-awake but not enough to get out of bed.
- Morin described hypervigilance processes operating during sleep but it's difficult to pin down particular content of threat due to the fact of sleep occurring.
- Attention biases are operating, but this is a touchy issue (the diagnosis means sufferers 100% believe they are awake and don't believe the sleep data)
- There is no sufficiently "awake" period to do the 20 min rule or restrict time in bed.
- Stimulus control therapy instructions of using bed only when sleepy and for sleep are complicated by clients believing "but I'm never sleepy".

So here are a few bits of evidence that someone diagnosed with Sleep State Misperception can consider to a) uncover any biases in thinking and attention, b) start a thought record like the one above, and c) attempt to clarify a mismatch between the poor sleep they feel and how others around them see it:

It may be sleep state misperception (& I sleep more than I think I do) if:

- I have a sleep study and disagree with the results on how long I slept, when the sleep technician has video and EEG data showing I was awake for 11 minutes when it felt like over an hour.

- I agree with my Fitbit when it says my hours of sleep are bad but I don't agree with it when it says my sleep hours are good. This is a selective bias, selecting only data that accords with my feelings and expectations.

- I recall that the things I was awake and thinking over carefully in my bed had some bizarre features so in retrospect were probably a dream.

- I hear from my partner that I was asleep and breathing regularly when I believed I was awake.

- I wake and notice I am on my back when I would never consciously fall asleep on my back (it probably happened during sleep);

- I continually ask myself "am I awake or asleep?" when I feel I'm really awake. The fact that I even have to ask this is evidence of a selective bias confirming my existing theory (It's pretty evident to most people when they are wide awake; they don't need to ask themselves if they are). The hypervigilance and frustration I feel when I doubt I am asleep can also be there in my sleep.

To test my fears: If I want to be sure I can always prove it to myself by keeping my eyes open and looking at the ceiling. Then I can truthfully say I'm awake. I'll try this as an behaviour experiment and see.

FITBIT RESULTS BIAS

A prominent example of thinking and attention bias around sleep is when we only believe our FITBIT or other sleep-measurement wearable if it says we didn't get much deep sleep, and not when it says we got a lot more deep sleep than we thought we did. If we believe our tiredness feelings instead of the Fitbit then that shows a bias towards a negative interpretation. It's also a thinking error we call "emotional reasoning" where we base our conclusions on what our emotions are telling us, not on the facts. Just see if you can catch this happening, as the starting point to questioning and overcoming biased sleep beliefs.

RETHINKING SLEEP SAFETY-SEEKING ACTIONS/ SAFEGUARDING

Scan this list of these sleep safety-seeking actions which make sense but backfire to create more sleep fears. Then take some time to think "Is there another way to look at this?".

SLEEPING IN UNTIL WHENEVER I CAN TO GET AT LEAST 8 HOURS SLEEP:

Sleeping in until whenever I can to get over 8 hours instead of keeping the same waking and rising time daily (to align with the sun rising, & to reset sleep wake schedule with the circadian rhythms)

Fear: I need more sleep! More sleep will make me feel better; I feel tired if I don't sleep in. I might get sick! My best sleep is 6-9am!

Another way to think of it:
1) Sure too little sleep is not good but too much – like over 9 hours a day, has health risks also. 7-7.5 hours is optimal for health. Also staying many more hours in bed can lead to fragmented, patchy sleep over time.
2) What is the evidence that I must have at least 8 hours of sleep every night? Is it because I think everyone else is sleeping 8 hours or more? What if I find that most of my friends don't sleep for 8 hours every night?
3) If this has been going on longterm, it is true I've got more sick? The people with the genetic defect who lose their capacity for slow wave sleep get very ill very quickly, and they all come from the same extended family in central America. Compared to them I'm not getting horribly sick.

The sad fact is, if you're looking for a continuous reward of 8 hours nightly sleep then you're looking in the wrong place. Initial use of sleep medications may shape the idea of "good sleep" to look like 6-8hours sedation. The user believes this is "deep sleep" all night because of the extended sedation, which is beyond what our physiology would ordinarily achieve. The truth is that real sleep is not consistently 8 solid sleep hours without fail every night. And it's certainly not 8 hours of *deep* sleep all night. Sleep quantity goes up and down, as your brain calibrates automatically whether you're in sleep deprivation or not, whether your homeostatic drive is significant, and whether or not it can afford to let you have a night without sleep so you can think about work or relationship stress.

What distinguishes "good" sleepers from insomnia sleepers is just that the unworried sleepers don't recall their waking periods during the night, while insomnia sufferers do. So unworried sleepers will tend to recall "Oh yeah, 8 hours from 10 until 6, as usual". The insomnia sufferers across multiple sleep studies are shown to get only 30 minutes average less sleep than "good" sleepers. But their recollection is that the waking periods went for many hours, or even all night, due to skewed sleep-wake perception.

DARKENING THE ROOM INSTEAD OF GETTING EARLY MORNING SUNLIGHT

Darkening my bedroom to avoid early morning sunlight (which would turn off my melatonin sleep hormone production and reset my circadian rhythm).

Fear: if I didn't sleep until 3am I need to sleep until 11am to get 8 hours!! My sleep onset is just broken, it doesn't work. I'm stuck being a night owl so I'll never hold down a day job.

Another way to think of it:
4) Was I looking on my phone/laptop until early morning to cope? Is it possible my melatonin production works fine but was just suppressed by blue light wave exposure?
5) Was I actually lying awake in bed with my eyes wide-awake open or closed? Is there any possibility I could have been asleep before 3am?
6) If I am able to sleep a consolidated 8 hours from 3-11am, what evidence is there that my sleep is broken. It just looks more like a delayed sleep-wake cycle, which is fixable with morning bright light and evening dim light.

SAFETY: HAVING NAPS DURING THE DAY TO GET ALL THE EXTRA SLEEP I CAN

Fear: I need all the sleep I can get, or I might get sick! (Instead of avoiding naps during the daytime if I have current insomnia to build up homeostatic pressure over the day's waking hours)

Another way to think of it:
1) Sure too little sleep – under 6 hours chronically - is not good but too much – like over 9 hours a day - has health risks also. More isn't better if it's over 9 hours. 7-7.5 hours sleep is optimal for health.
2) a 20-30 min nap is okay if I have no insomnia, but is my napping during the day taking away from my sleep at night? Since I have insomnia problems and a big 1 hour wake period at 2 am can I try to go without the nap to consolidate my sleep at night? And generating energy during the day by going for a walk instead of sleeping? I don't have to drive at work and when I didn't nap previously I was able to stay awake and do things in the afternoon instead. I'm now cancelling social things on weekend afternoons so it's starting to affect my social life.
3) If this has been going on awhile have I actually been getting more sick? What does my doctor say about this?

GOING TO BED EVEN IF I'M NOT SLEEPY

Going to bed even if I feel completely awake and alert. (Instead of going to bed only when sleepy, to strengthen association of my bed with sleep and reduce my chances of bed being associated with wakefulness).

Fear: I keep to a regular bedtime wind-down routine – it should work! I'm doing all the right things, I don't want to waste the wind-down, and I don't want to have to go through it again! Maybe if I'm resting in bed, it's as good as sleeping? (Instead of only going to bed when I feel sleepy to associate your bed with sleep & strengthen this paired association over time).

STAYING IN BED EVEN IF I'M WIDE AWAKE AT NIGHT

Staying in bed if I just can't sleep at night. (Instead of getting out of bed if unable to sleep within 20 minutes and spending quiet time in another room until I have sleepiness signs again to untrain a conditioned association of my bed with wakefulness.)

Fear: I need to sleep! If I get up then I'll have no hope of getting back to sleep! Maybe if I'm resting in bed, it's as good as sleeping?

Another way to think of it:
No one said this was going to be easy, but if I can persevere with this, especially under difficult conditions, then I'll ultimately get better sleep out of it.

Reaching 90% sleep efficiency will involve frustration and distress tolerance. But the rewards are great.

Yes, we are restricting time in bed to increase sleep efficiency. It sounds counterintuitive at first, but when I really think about it, I'll get more sleep in less time, less fragmented sleep and less frustrated wakefulness during the night. I won't be spending hours in exhausting worry and rumination, which is a relief.

It feels right to spend more time in bed to get more sleep, but that sleep safety-seeking behaviour has contributed to my present insomnia problem.

SLEEPING IN UNTIL WHENEVER I CAN TO GET MORE SLEEP:
Instead of using bright light to train back natural waking time if more than 4 hours after dawn, set alarm for natural waking time & get exposure to bright light. Then set alarm for 30 minutes earlier on each subsequent day (and don't return to sleep after alarm sounds) until goal waking & rising time is achieved, and early morning sunlight exposure occurs.

Fear: if I don't sleep until midday I will become sleep deprived.

Another way to think of it:

It's costing me to sleep until midday. Many people have trained their delayed sleep-wake problem back to an earlier rising time. There's no reason why I can't also. In fact, no-one gets sleep onset guaranteed, the only place we can train from is backwards from bright sunlight in the morning – the handbrake on sleep cycle delays.

At least my sleep is already consolidated – I get a block of 7 hours a day. If I get fewer hours a night at first I will make it up a few days later as my brain recognizes I'm in mild sleep deprivation. But I may not even get sleep deprived since I'm marching my waking time back gradually at just 30 minutes earlier every day.   I'll just pick my days off to start the training.

USING MEDICATION AFTER MISSING A NIGHT'S SLEEP WHEN I DON'T USUALLY USE IT

Another way to think of it:

I can try interpreting the situation by looking at my homeostatic sleep pressure over several days. When I have a night of 2 hours sleep next time I'll look at the night before it. Looking back over the sleep diary there may be was a longer sleep duration the night prior.

Many people have conditioned a pattern of alternating "good" and "bad" sleeps when they seek help for insomnia. I could justifiably frame this happening as the circadian and homeostatic drives working just fine. My brain assesses that I want to stay alert for threats a full night (same part of my brain that would've been alert for predators 30,000 years ago) and gives me the leeway based on the adequate sleep I experienced the night before. If I had no sleep the night before my brain would be much less likely to allow me another night off sleep; the adenosine sleep-inducer levels in the brain would have been too great.

NOTE: In an insomnia clinic many people present with a conditioned pattern of 2 nights poor sleep. Unfortunately, just as their homeostatic drive would have overtaken them on the third night, they have taken sleep medication in a desperate panic to avoid a third sleepless night. This means, when they sleep solidly on that third night, they then attribute the good sleep to the medication rather than their own sleep self-regulation. They think the sleep couldn't possibly be the result of their brain's sleep processes ("my sleep was broken for two nights, who knows how long it could have gone on!") and instead renew their trust in the medication. Not getting the chance to see homeostatic pressure would have worked means the fears and distrust in their own ability to sleep were confirmed.

Another way to think of it.

I can consider the evidence of Randy Gardner, who is still the World Guinness Book of Records holder for sleep deprivation, and his record dates from over 40 years ago. Many have tried since but no one was able to match his sleep deprivation record of 11 days and nights. What's interesting about this case was he didn't need the equivalent time to make up an estimated 77 hour sleep deficit (if he slept around 7 hours per night); he only needed 3 recovery nights (and was awake during the days) of 15 hours (first night), 10.5 hours (second night) and back to near-normal with 9 hours (third night).

But what's most intriguing is how his brain self-regulated to give him almost doubled the amount of deep, slow-wave sleep, almost double the amount of REM dream sleep, and almost halved stage 1 and 2 light sleep over those three recovery nights. He had no control over how his brain self-regulated the sleep, and it suggests the importance of deep sleep and dream sleep that these predominated over light sleep during the recovery sleeps.

What's reassuring about Randy Gardner's results for me/my sleep:

Try to avoid alcohol or prescription sleep medications before bed if you haven't been using them yet. If dependent on sleep medications establish a tapering regime to reduce alongside CBT program (goal is to understand attributing sleep to substances, and preparedness to learn sleep habits & calm CNS on own vs depend on sedative & hypnotic medications to get to sleep).

Example of fears: But I'm not getting enough sleep! I need to get something from my doctor to help me sleep – I can't do it myself!"

What to try: You may be right, but just to be sure, gather some evidence over 2 weeks with a sleep diary which you can take to your doctor (see the 2-week Sleep diary). Or you can collect Fitbit sleep wearable data over 2 weeks and review that. What if you were to disagree with the Fitbit over the amount of deep sleep it says you've had?

Try using a thought record (below) for this evidence-gathering:

My negative (fearful, frustrated) thoughts about sleep	How these thoughts make me feel	Evidence For fearful thought ie cost **will be big** if poor sleep	Evidence against fearful thought ie cost **will not be big** if poor sleep	Balanced, alternative thought	How I feel now
My sleep is so bad I….					
If this goes on….					

Don't forget to add in any evidence from other people that might come up. You might find some evidence by just noticing sleep cues overtaking you:

"It is sleep cues if I feel heavy head, droopy eyes. Heavy eyelids. Losing place on the page. Rereading lines. Watching a film and realizing I missed a bit of the scene because of a micro sleep. Suddenly becoming aware I was snoring, or my partner tells me I was."

GOING TO THE TOILET MULTIPLE TIMES BEFORE BED, RELATED TO INSOMNIA
Going to the toilet a number of times close to bedtime is an understandable sleep safeguarding action. No one wants to be woken too early from sleep by bladder fullness messages. Especially if you're scared you won't get back to sleep again.

Certainly if you have a history of UTI, diabetes Types I or II, kidney stones, or cystitis then get a thorough medical checkup to find any medical cause of excess urinating. But most insomnia sufferers will know if it's been going on a long time and isn't medically-caused but is instead more sleep anxiety-related. Then it is likely to have become a conditioned reflex as part of your insomnia picture.

Questions to ask yourself to clarify if it's anxiety or a physiological problem:
Does it happen every night and it's been happening a long time now?
Do I notice that there's no obstruction or difficulty peeing (such as with a UTI), I've just been too focused on completely emptying my bladder so I can get to sleep?
Do my worst anxieties ultimately relate to sleep, not to a UTI? (if UTI's rare for me?)
Do I notice that anxiety, not the need to pee, builds again after peeing as I lie awake in bed scanning for bladder pressure?
Do I notice the anxiety won't go away until I have to go to the toilet again to reduce anxiety?
Am I noticing over time I feel more anxiety about sleep with all the toilet visits, not less?
Am I noticing thoughts like "Just to be safe, one last pee; then I'll be able to sleep"?
Am I noticing I do other sleep safeguarding behaviours like not drinking water many hours before bed to try to guarantee my bladder won't be full during the night?

WHAT HAPPENS WITH EXCESSIVE URINATING
Two things happen because of too-frequent urinating in insomnia:
Physically, your bladder capacity shrinks over time, so you get messages more frequently that it's full compared to when it held more capacity.
Psychologically your anxiety and your doubts will build over time as you simultaneously overvalue and distrust your brain's sleep processes. Your attention will keep going back to your bladder sensations, constantly assessing bladder pressure and looking for threats to your sleep.

Treatment: The antidote to this sleep-safeguarding is to:
1) First a checkup and tests with your medical practitioner, to rule out UTI.
2) If your doctor endorses it, start Bladder Training, to build up capacity by waiting for longer before you urinate. You can train your bladder to hold out for longer before sending urgent messages. Many women's hospitals offer this training to women after childbirth and menopause (in menopause lowered oestrogen level lead to urinating more)

3) Do Kegel exercises (will be part of a post-childbirth hospital training course also, after childbirth weakens and stretches the pelvic floor muscles and urethra) which will strengthen the pelvic floor muscles to increase control and confidence about holding on.
4) Drink less caffeine or alcohol drinks close to bedtime, (these are diuretics and flush more water out of your system).
5) If anxiety about sleep is the main issue, look at ways to manage your anxiety. Read over the other reassuring information about your brain's ability to regulate sleep and see if it has some effect on your anxiety:
6) Consider this evidence also: Slow-wave sleep signals to your body to make a hormone (ADH) which tells your body to hold onto fluid until you wake up.

(If you have Sleep Apnoea, however, it interrupts your breathing and stops your body from getting to the stage where it produces ADH hormone. Plus blood doesn't get enough oxygen, which is a trigger for your kidneys to get rid of water. *This is another important health reason to get any snoring or gasping during sleep checked out with your doctor and then an overnight sleep study*).

SQUEEZING YOUR EYES CLOSED TO TRY TO GET BACK TO SLEEP

Even tightly closing your eyes in bed signals that you aren't able to control or force sleep. Once you become aware that you can't sleep, closing your eyes is part of sleep *effort*. It's part of trying to make sleep happen, rather than just let it happen. It just increases preoccupation with the ongoing poor sleep, and all the bad consequences (health and next day functioning) that could result. It increases frustration that you can't control your brain in its sleep processes.

The best thing to do: accept you aren't sleeping and try this action:
1) Open your eyes to confirm you are not sleeping. Too many times people experience uncertainty and sleep state misperception because with their eyes closed they may have been drifting into sleep. This is annoying for them because they *felt* strongly that they weren't asleep, but didn't have enough evidence to prove it to themselves.
2) This is part of the paradoxical intention experiment at Glasgow University where insomnia sufferers were instructed to keep their eyes open and try to stay awake, compared with others who were instructed to try to go to sleep. Those keeping their eyes open and staring at the ceiling ended up with less sleep effort and more sleep hours compared to the unchanged sleep hours of those trying to sleep.
3) Keeping your eyes open has the powerful effect of changing your expectations about sleep, and reducing sleep performance anxiety (wanting sleep but fearing that you can't get to sleep).

WEIGHTED BLANKETS

The evidence of effectiveness is varied, and it's difficult to do Randomised Controlled Trials on weighted blankets (blankets with a grid of stitched squares filled with small plastic or glass beads, said to "hug" the sleeper, with up to 25 pounds inhibiting restless movement. The sleeper with insomnia can feel more secure and less anxious, so sleep more soundly. Overheating can be an issue with weighted blankets, and increased core body temperature does affect ability to get to sleep and stay asleep. Also some people experience claustrophobia under a weighted blanket, which will increase heart rate and core body temperature, making it hard to achieve or maintain sleep.

LEARNED HELPLESSNESS
Learned helplessness happens when we try repeatedly to problem-solve insomnia yet become more hypervigilant and sleepless for our efforts. We begin to feel helpless because we see no way to influence the sleep outcome and we become conditioned to expect wakeful suffering night after night. We simply give up. This apathy and loss of motivation can ultimately generate depression. Learned helplessness is particularly a risk once tolerance to sleep medications develops, and attributions have shifted from our own personal agency to the medication taking care of sleep. This is why behaviour experiments to test expectations about sleep are so important: we get to relearn that we're not helpless if we moderate our expectations and allow the brain to get on with its job without trying repeatedly to control it.

THE BEST SLEEP AID: NON-JUDMENTAL STANCE/ACCEPTANCE
Using mindfulness, present moment awareness, nonjudgmental stance and open acceptance of our brain's sleep regulation processes, we will cope better with sleep ups and downs. Mindfulness, not just about where your attention is directed or placed, but about your *willingness* to shelve judgment on your brain's sleep regulation. If you can experience some curiosity about the insomnia experience, it will help you put judgment aside, and make it easier to tolerate the wakefulness.

If we take tinnitus coping as an example, tinnitus sufferers who can allow some curiosity about even 2 hours of being able to ignore tinnitus, or not alerting to it constantly, actually start to habituate, and desensitise to the aversive signals. They hold off judgment of threat. They feel surprise and curiosity when they find they could ignore it a bit more – first for 2 hours, then 2 days, then 2 weeks. Opening up their attention rewards them with more curiosity about what the desensitising and habituating brain is capable of.

If the tinnitus patient can notice "There are actually things I can do to cope/make it better" there will be an increase in feelings of agency and mastery (ie believing that you can influence outcomes, when you previously felt helpless). This works exactly the same way for insomnia sufferers. Just bringing attention to small improvements or surprises, in behaviour habits and expectation, can make an insomnia sufferer feel capable of increased coping and mastery. This will go a long way toward helplessness feelings and fears of sleep uncontrollability and unpredictability.

CHAPTER 9   INSOMNIA, WORRY AND RUMINATION
Conditioning bed as a signal to worry – functions of worry – positive & negative beliefs about worry - worry logging and worry session with Problem solving- Understanding Rumination – Rumination Cues Action exercise

Worrying is the main activity that people describe doing when they lie in bed hoping that sleep will come, and getting frustrated and anxious about it. It usually starts off as worry about work, family, the future, finances, security, safety. Then as more sleep is lost over multiple nights, it extends to worry about the costs of sleep loss. So, not only the original worry, but also consequences of sleep deprivation worries! Health consequences, job consequences, parenting or relationship consequences, and also the sheer unpredictability and uncontrollability of sleep.

WORRY GETS CONDITIONED TO YOUR BED AT NIGHT
Over time the worry gets conditioned to the bed environment, and even to a particular time of the night. A conditioned association of the bed to wakefulness and worry, at a reliable time, almost every night. And as we've already seen, you can't just *think* your way out of a conditioned insomnia response. Your central nervous system is too programmed to get you into problem solving mode in the middle of the night.

WORRY IS FUNCTIONAL
And this is the hard thing to accept about worry. That it functions to protect us from future harm. Let's think about how *sensible* it is to worry. How adaptive (20,000 years ago your worrying ancestors would've woken with raised spears at the slightest rustle of the approaching predator. Meanwhile the deep-sleeping people in the next cave would've been mauled). Never mind about how exhausting and tiring it is. If you're a good problem solver then you've already got a history of getting out of scrapes or fixing work problems. Well, worry can be seen as mental problem solving to anticipate negative future events and then prevent them from happening.

It's not too far from writing checklists of "to do" items, which are also designed to prevent stress and last-minute catastrophes. Worry only becomes unhelpful when it is frequent, with multiple feared events warranting constant monitoring, and hard to control or dismiss.

So given how inherently adaptive it is, you can see why we hold *positive* beliefs about worrying:
For example: "Worry motivates me to find solutions – I don't care if it's bad news, I want to see it coming so I can feel more in control". "Worrying helps me avoid or prevent bad things, and at least prepares me for the worst if I can't control the bad thing".

DON'T GET ANGRY AT YOURSELF FOR WORRYING
This is why you can't get angry at yourself for worrying. No matter what your negative beliefs of how exhausting and energy-sapping it is, worry functions to help you anticipate future harm, and avoid it. It's all about taking responsibility, and with worry you're doing the best you can to be a careful, conscientious person who cares about preventing harm. What can be better than that?

What keeps my worry going?

Negative beliefs about worry *eg worry exhausts me, harms my health*	
Positive beliefs about worry *eg Worry helps me anticipate & avoid danger*	
Avoidance *eg if I avoid all risk I can stay safe & not regret things*	
Thought control *eg I will try hard to blank my mind of any bad thoughts*	
Refusal to accept uncertainty *eg I need to know what's going to happen at all times*	

KEEPING IT CONTAINED

So worry only becomes truly draining when it's entrenched meaninglessness, when you know you're in a conditioned habit of worrying frequently and excessively about the smallest things, that don't ever eventuate anyway. When you are constantly overestimating the likelihood of threat and overestimating how severe the impact. Avoiding more and more to avoid all foreseeable risk and stay safe, or feeling so overwhelmed by the uncontrollability and uncertainty of the future so that problems that *are* solveable get unnoticed.

This is where a worries log and worries session can help.

Please make copies of this worry recording log following so you can get into practice at dumping your worries on to the page. If your brain gets practice at thinking of this as "external storage" it may be more able to "let go" of the worries and let you resume sleep during the night.

WORRIES LOG: Complete during daytime worry session, NOT at bedtime or when waking during night		
Write down worry content	Type of worry: is it....?	Am I doing...?
Eg *what if I ruin the talk tomorrow and get sacked?*	o Concrete current problem needing immediate attention Vs o Hypothetical "what if....?" problem	o Constructive problem solving Vs o Pointless speculation
	o Concrete current problem needing immediate attention Vs o Hypothetical "what if....?" problem	o Constructive problem solving vs o Pointless speculation
	o Concrete current problem needing immediate attention Vs o Hypothetical "what if....?" problem	o Constructive problem solving Vs o Pointless speculation

LETTING GO OF NIGHT-TIME WORRY

By the way, it's best not to have this intimidating white page on your bedside table; this one is for filling in only upon waking in the morning with just a few worry keywords or a one-line prompt to recall your worry at the later worry session. This worry session will preferably be at the same place (eg kitchen table) and same time (eg 8am or 6pm) "worry spot" where you will now train your worry to be conditioned. On your bedside table just have ready one of those little notepads that come in children's party packs or lolly bags. This is deliberate because we want to lower any expectation on you to write something perfectly precise or detailed at 2am.

Soon after waking, before you start to get frustrated at keeping a reminder bobbing in your mind for tomorrow morning, write down 2 key words only. This is also a great exercise in trusting your memory, because you're trusting that these 2 key words will be the launchpad tomorrow morning for the complex associations that branch off them. To scrawl 2 words down you don't even need the bedside light on. Then drop the pen and close your eyes and experiment with capturing a dream fragment or wiggling your toes to see if your brain lets go of the worry and lets you resume sleep. Just doing this is already priming your brain to expect that bed isn't the place to "hold onto" worries. If it doesn't work, (and allowing it not to is crucial, incidentally) and you're still worrying about the same thing 20 minutes later, you'll then need to consider getting out of bed to do the "20 minute rule" as discussed already.

COPING STATEMENTS AT 2AM

Just gently encourage yourself to let it go with "I can't think clearly at 2am, I will solve it better in just 4-5 hours, in my regular worry session, when I CAN think clearly".
If it's clearly "what if...?" pointless speculation about imagined future catastrophe, then try saying "this is a "what if?" thought again, these are always about catastrophes that just don't seem to happen. Even if I write it down now I know I'll think it's ridiculous tomorrow morning. Just like last time."

MY INSOMNIA WORRIES LOG (Adapted from Edelman) -SPECIFICS:

1. I'll complete this during a daytime worry session, <u>not </u>at bedtime or during waking periods at night. The goal is to condition worry away from my bed, and away from 2am.

2. Have a small notepad on my bedside table; when half-awake *leave light off*, pick up pen & write down 2 keywords only on notepad. Then drop pen & think "It's in external storage now; I can let go 'til (8am worry session)". Then *test* if my brain will let me return to sleep.

3. Allow lowered sleep expectations if I have a *conditioned* worry period at 2am. I may need to leave bed to reassociate bed with sleep if I become more awake at this time. I accept this is part of unconditioning the habit. I will do something calming in the other room, not complex problem solving, which I want to condition to daytime instead.

4. I should actually *do* the worry session in the daytime (same time, same place) to effectively condition the worry away from my bed at 2am. And satisfy my brain I have set aside time to problem-solve properly.

During my daytime worry session log worry content here:	Type of worry: is it:	Am I doing:
Eg *what if I ruin the talk tomorrow and get sacked?*	○ concrete current problem that needs my immediate attention ○ hypothetical problem (what if...?!)	○ Problem solving? ○ Pointless speculation about future?
	○ concrete current problem that needs my immediate attention ○ hypothetical problem (what if...?!)	○ Problem solving? ○ Pointless speculation about future?

Review after 3 weeks daily practice:	Log useful-why?	Log not useful-why?

Worries log: Before & After

Am I finding a pattern of overestimating danger/threat after the event passes?

Before the event What do I fear will happen?	**After the event** What actually happened?
Review after 3 weeks practice: If more than 4 examples in 1 week (of catastrophizing):	Do I have a bias for overestimating threat that is affecting my sleep? Questions: How likely? how severe will it really be?

TOMORROW'S WORRY SESSION

The next morning you transfer the key words from your little notepad to the worries log above, and then set it aside for your worry/problem solving session later that day. If it's just checklisting, all well and good. You can add it to your "to-do" list for the day. If it's worry content, you've already started training your brain to shift "worry time" from the night to the daytime. This "shift" needs practice, by the way. You can't force your brain to suddenly start worrying localised to 8am daytime. You need to gently nudge it forward into the day, and reinforce that new learning *every day* to make it stick. If you don't do the worry session, your brain will opt for "well I still need to problem solve this important future threat, and 2am is the only quiet time with no distractions, so it will have to be complex thinking at 2am again".

Very often, however, the all-important key words that people write down during the night, that *"Absolutely Must Be Recalled"* in the morning, turn out next morning to be trivial and not worth the sleeplessness. People are incredulous that they gave such emotional weight to these worries during the night. But then again, surely we're not expecting to think rationally when waking at 2am? It's important to remind ourselves "I can't think clearly now at 2am, my brain wants to sleep. I will solve this at my worry session tomorrow."

During the worry session next day, try asking yourself these questions:

Worry session: 20 mins in daytime	
What's the most worrying thing in this? (core worry)	
What are all the solutions I can think of? Brainstorm – no solution off-limits	
What's the most sensible solution to try out?	
Is my worry realistic? How likely is it?	
If it happens how bad would it really be?	
Does this really matter to me?	
Am I just worrying out of habit, or do I really care about this?	
Is it solvable or preventable? (problem-solve)	
Or not in my control? (Acceptance)	

RUMINATION
Raking over past regrets, injustices, guilt - "coulda, shoulda, woulda" - self-critical helplessness - Rumination cues Action exercise

Rumination is related to worry and often interchangeable with it during the night. It is often described as raking over past regrets and injustices; things that we or others should've done, could've done, would've done, that can't be changed. It's normal, and to some extent everyone dwells on things because it overlaps with problem-solving and learning from the past to correct or avoid things in the future.

So thinking about what we could've done better can be helpful; especially if we reach a solution & put it into action. Also, most of the time and for most people, rumination is time-limited: it stops when the problem is solved. The main problem with it is becoming preoccupied with something and feeling unable to get it out of our minds, such that we are overwhelmed by self-critical helplessness and distress.

What's wrong with Rumination as learning?
- rumination tends to focus on causes & consequences instead of solutions. "What did I do to ruin my sleep?" & "Will my sleep ever get better?" instead of "How do I make my sleep better?"
- Rumination tends to focus on what has gone wrong & lead to self-blame and further negative thinking.
- When attention stays on rumination activity it generally maintains helplessness & depression.
- Rumination tends to foster inactivity & avoidance of problem-solving

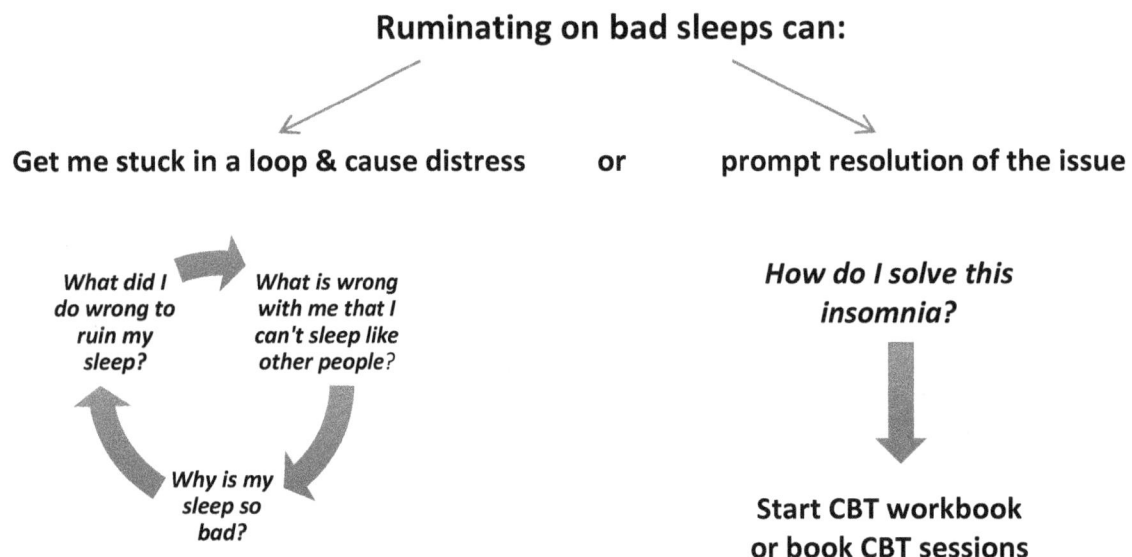

Ruminating on bad sleeps can:

Get me stuck in a loop & cause distress   or   **prompt resolution of the issue**

What did I do wrong to ruin my sleep? → *What is wrong with me that I can't sleep like other people?* → *Why is my sleep so bad?* →

How do I solve this insomnia?

Start CBT workbook or book CBT sessions

WHEN RUMINATION PREVENTS PROBLEM SOLVING

To stop rumination preventing your problem solving, you can learn to gain control over it. And the first step to gaining control over rumination is to recognise it when it happens. You know you're ruminating if:

- You're stuck thinking about distressing thoughts, feelings, or situations.
- The process of raking over and over something is not helping you feel more hopeful, or less self-critical.
- The process of thinking has not helped you to solve a problem.

The 3-point rule for recognizing rumination

When you catch yourself ruminating stop and ask yourself these three questions:

1. Am I making progress toward solving my sleep problem?
2. Do I understand more about my sleep problem or my feelings about it?
3. Do I feel less self-critical or less depressed about my sleep than before I started thinking about this?

If the answer to these questions is no, assume you're ruminating and then try this training strategy below.

RUMINATION CUES ACTION STRATEGY

Unlikely as it seems, you can teach yourself to use ruminating as a cue to get active. You can use a strategy called "**rumination cues action**". A cue is something that prompts you to behave in a certain way. For example, a red stop sign is a cue to slow down a car and stop. Unfortunately, if you regularly ruminate, then many things in your life would cue you to engage in this. And ruminating itself has likely become a cue to further ruminating. But that will change with 3 simple steps:

1. First you need to catch when you ruminate and notice ways it has cost you or your sleep.
2. Then you spend some time practising attention shifts until you find it easier to direct your attention *toward a valued action*, rather than *running from an aversive action*.
3. Then you practice both catching your rumination and using it to redirect your attention.

Exercise 1: Monitoring Rumination

Over the next week, see if you can recognise and label rumination when it occurs. When you do recognise it, say to yourself, "This is rumination" or "I'm ruminating again!" You will be surprised at how powerful it can be to simply increase your awareness of your actions. You will start to find that labelling rumination helps you to control it.

Use the space below to monitor ruminating when it happens. In the first column, record the situation in which you observed yourself ruminating. In the 2nd column record what you were ruminating about. In the 3rd column identify the consequence/cost of ruminating. See the example of recording rumination below to guide you.

	Situation	Rumination	Consequence/Cost
e.g.	Driving home after work	"I shouldn't have said that! I'm an idiot."	Felt more stupid, depressed. Almost drove through a stop sign.
1.			
2.			
3.			
4.			

Exercise 2: Paying Attention

Over the next couple of days, practice attending mindfully, in the present moment, to your experience in situations where you might normally ruminate. Below is space for you to write down the situations you are in and what you gave your full attention to:

Day	Situation	I attended to…
e.g after lunch	Sitting at my work computer	What I was reading, feeling my posture as I was sitting & the warm air, my steady breathing, sounds in the room and outside.

Exercise 3: Rumination Cues Action Worksheet

Now after practicing the first 2 exercises try combining them together as below. So catch the rumination and then cue in redirection to mindful activity in the present moment:

	Situation	Catch the Rumination: "I'm ruminating!"	Cues	Action/Shift Attention to:
e.g.	Walking back to my car after work	"I shouldn't have said that! I'm an idiot."… "Hey, I'm ruminating!"	→	1. Listen to sounds around me (birds) 2. Smells around me 3. Feeling of walking 4. Sights around me (people, trees, sky)
1.			→	
2.			→	
3.			→	
4.			→	
5.			→	

CHAPTER 10   CBT EXPERIMENTS WITH SLEEP SAFEGUARDING & SLEEP EFFORT: UNLEARNING HABITS THROUGH BEHAVIOUR CHANGE EXPERIMENTS

CBT behavior-change experiment benefits. Rigid 8hr sleep rule experiment. Worry Logging experiment. Surveying other sleepers experiment. Thought-blanking experiment. "Leaky battery" energy-generating experiment. Nasal spray experiment. Paradoxical intention experiment.

Behavioural experiments in InsomniaCBT have the power to disconfirm our existing unhelpful thinking and provide evidence for new, more helpful beliefs and expectations. "Learning by doing" experiments trigger more thinking, feeling and behavior change than just verbal interventions. The simultaneous change in thinking, feeling and acting comes through experiential learning, heightened emotional processing, multisensory encoding of experiences in memory at different levels, learning through reflection, and practicing new plans and actions.

As discussed earlier, CBT stimulus control strategies are the key experiments that change insomnia habits and expectations. Try this experiment if you have rigid rules on the necessity of 8 hours sleep per night due to fears of health or daytime functioning impacts. Here's an example of how to record your 3-week sleep consolidation experiment:

EXPERIMENT: Consolidating sleep to test rigid 8hr sleep rule (adapted from Ree & Harvey, 2004)				
Initial belief	Alternative belief	experiment	result	reflection
I need at least 8 hrs sleep to function ok in the day; I must spend 8+ hours in bed.. Under 8 hours is dangerous for health.	I can probably cope quite well after 6-7 hours sleep. I don't need exactly 8 hrs every night – a range is normal.	Restrict sleep to 6.5 hrs by going to bed 1 hour later. Stay awake by going to dinner with friends	I actually coped fine with 6.5hrs sleep; in fact I got 6 hrs sleep 4 days earlier and was surprised at how well I functioned at work. Also found after going out with friends my mood the next day was much better.	My health & my coping ability is just the same with a range of 6-8 hours. The worry was the worst part. I don't need to have 8hrs every night to cope. Is good for me to go out with friends, I can defocus from sleep & it actually gets better.
Initial belief	Alternative belief	experiment	result	reflection

People with conditioned insomnia and worry periods during the night may understandably feel doubtful about "training" their worry away from the bed and away from the middle of the night. Just trialling the worry log and worry session daily for 3 weeks surprises people in its effectiveness.   What is there to lose? Here's an example of how to do the experiment:

EXPERIMENT:Doing Worry Logging & Worry Session for 3 weeks				
Initial belief	Alternative belief	experiment	result	reflection
I can't control my worries	*I'm too busy to problem-solve during the day so I end up doing it at 2am.* *If I do a worry session at 5pm & problem-solve then I may be able to control when I worry better*	*Use worry log for 3 weeks to record my worries & do daily worry session at 5pm to problem solve them; to reduce 2am waking & worrying.*	*The worry session showed I can train my worry to 5pm and let it go at 2am, as long as I do it daily. . Worry log showed me I catastrophise about work*	*Doing 5pm worry & problem solving session helped my sleep.Writing worries on paper & decent problem-solving time means I'm generally calmer & I catastrophise less.*
Initial belief	Alternative belief	experiment	result	reflection

SURVEYING OTHER SLEEPERS WHEN I BELIEVE I'M ALONE IN GETTING LESS THAN 8HR SLEEP

EXPERIMENT: Survey other sleepers to see if I am only one with less than 8 hours (adapted from Ree & Harvey, 2004)				
Initial belief	Alternative belief	experiment	result	reflection
Everyone else gets 8 hours and they're not tired; my sleep is defective	*Other people don't get 8 hrs every night; it's not a realistic expectation*	*Collaborate on survey for 20 others: how long to fall asleep, hours estimated, waking episodes + duration; ever tired in a.m.*	*Others also get less than 8 hrs and function well; all have less sleep when stressed; some tired after lunch even with 8hrs- didn't expect this*	*Quantity is not equal to quality; since asking others I've seen myself that I can have better energy on 6hr sleeps than on >8hr sleeps; I'm no different to others really.*
Initial belief	Alternative belief	experiment	result	reflection

THOUGHT SUPPRESSION EXPERIMENT

This one is quick and easy to do and helps us understand the futility of trying to suppress or blank out worrying thoughts when awake at night.

EXPERIMENT: test thought-blanking effectiveness (adapted from Ree & Harvey, 2004)				
Initial belief	Alternative belief	experiment	result	reflection
Worrying at night is dangerous and I need to blank out my mind and blank my thoughts.	Trying to blank out thoughts is not possible, it will create more fight-flight and worry that I can't control my mind.	For 1 minute concentrate very hard on not thinking about a pink elephant	Found that the more I tried to blank out the image the more it filled my mind.	It will be better for my sleep if I save myself the effort of trying to blank my mind of all thoughts. The job of my brain is to generate thoughts, after all. I'll try the worry log instead.
Initial belief	Alternative belief	experiment	result	reflection

DAYTIME EXPERIMENT TO TEST FEARS ABOUT POOR SLEEP & INADEQUATE ENERGY

EXPERIMENT: My energy is like a leaky battery, must conserve it (adapted from Ree & Harvey, 2004)				
Initial belief	Alternative belief	experiment	result	reflection
My energy is like a leaky battery and I need to conserve it because I can only replenish it through sleep.	Maybe my energy is not that finite, maybe it's more like an elastic band, with more stretch than I expect.	Test 1 day conserving energy vs 1 day creating and using up energy. Rate tiredness and coping levels after each day then compare both days' results.	I actually had more energy and felt I coped better by creating energy with walking and socialising, compared to feeling very tired the day I conserved energy and basically withdrew.	My energy and my mood are helped by daytime activity and not avoiding, vs conserving energy & isolating myself. And my sleep is actually better after exercising during the day!
Initial belief	Alternative belief	experiment	result	reflection

DECONGESTANT NASAL SPRAY EXPERIMENT

EXPERIMENT: See if reducing nasal spray reliance worsens my sleep (adapted from Ree & Harvey, 2004)

Initial belief	Alternative belief	experiment	result	reflection
I must be on nasal decongestant spray all my life to get the sleep I need.	*I'm waking with rebound nasal congestion at 3am & panicking. Plain saline nasal spray can work just as well without the rebound nasal congestion. My GP says I should trial this; GP & spray manufacturer said to only use short term.*	Gradually reduce number of decongestant sprays per day over 2 weeks and replace with plain saline spray.	*Rebound nasal congestion bad at first but using saline spray felt reassuring & I panicked less because I changed them gradually. 3am waking stopped after my anxiety about breathing reduced.*	*Am less focused on my nose, my breathing & sleep now. Don't need 100% clear nasal passages to get to sleep. Actually need less sprays now I'm not panicking. .*
Initial belief	Alternative belief	experiment	result	reflection

Glasgow University paradoxical intention experiment, targeting sleep expectations:

EXPERIMENT: See if trying to stay awake at night worsens my sleep (adapted from Ree & Harvey, 2004)

Initial belief	Alternative belief	experiment	result	reflection
I must get to sleep doing everything possible	*Maybe trying to stay awake will reduce the pressure I put on myself to sleep*	Spend 4 nights in a row with eyes open, staring at ceiling (not electronic device) & trying to stay awake	*Actually got more hours sleep when trying to stay awake and stare at ceiling! Didn't expect this at all.*	*I have less sleep effort and less performance anxiety about sleep by changing my 'should' expectations about sleep.*
Initial belief	Alternative belief	experiment	result	reflection

1 MONTH REVIEW OF BEHAVIOUR CHANGE EXPERIMENTS:

After doing these behaviour change experiments over the past month I learned:	
Experiment(s) done:	My impressions: (what changed/what didn't) & surprises

CHAPTER 11   YOUR VALUES WILL HELP YOU OVERCOME INSOMNIA

Let's start by exploring how the quality of your life has been affected by insomnia. In what ways has this happened? Write down a few areas where insomnia has changed your choices and actions.

Ways my quality of life is reduced by insomnia	What I'd be doing if I didn't have insomnia
Daytime: eg, too tired to meet up with old friends	Daytime: Walk with friend at 7am on beach. Meet friends for lunch.
Night-time: Eg, Haven't been to a party in years due to 9.30pm bedtime	Night-time: Go to concert with my friends

Now think about these questions: Am I conserving energy by cancelling appointments and being less active? Only to find that I am 1) still tired and low in energy, and 2) resentful I'm missing out on life?

This is where a values review can help you overcome insomnia. A values review?
Well, we generally don't like to stop doing our safeguarding or safety-seeking behaviours when we have insomnia -that's why they're called safety-seeking after all. From using prescription medications to spending extended hours in bed trying to sleep, we're only doing them to try to bring about sleep and safeguard sleep. Unfortunately, as we've already found, the safety behaviours backfire to create more hypervigilance and insomnia. And that means more time in bed spent sleepless and less quality of life.

But just knowing about backfiring safety behaviours doesn't seem helpful: "how do I not try to sleep? Are you saying all these good sleep strategies – the commonsense ones like going to bed early every night and giving myself more time in bed for sleep – make this worse? Why would I restrict my time in bed?"

Well there's no doubt in the clinical research that the core behaviour change strategies work: of keeping the same waking time daily, early morning sunlight exposure, going to bed when sleepy and using the bed only for sleep, and restricting time in bed to your actual sleep time.

But all these are hard to do when we 1) overvalue sleep and 2) try too hard to make it happen. It's hard to reconcile the idea of LETTING sleep happen when you want to problem-solve proactively and MAKE sleep happen.

The safety-seeking behaviour of spending more time in bed makes intuitive sense.

(I know how to get more sleep! Spend more time in bed!") So the idea of reducing time in bed to consolidate sleep and reassociate bed with sleep seems crazy.

Glasgow University's Colin Espie talks about "the thin line" between commitment (to overcome insomnia) and unproductive effort. And there *is* a fine line between being motivated to overcome insomnia, and being too preoccupied by it, to the point where sleep becomes effortful and you start to distrust in your brain's ability to self-regulate sleep.

INTUITIVE REASONS TO STAY IN BED
Even if we don't like laying awake in frustration in bed for hours on end, we reframe it to have a positive meaning ("at least I'm resting even if I'm not sleeping"). After all, better the devil you know, right? Outside of bed seems way more uncertain. Staying in bed might be grim but at least it's familiar.

So here's the difficult question: What could motivate us to do something as counter-intuitive as restricting our time in bed? For example, going out with friends some nights instead of keeping to a rigid early bedtime; getting out of bed to go for a morning walk instead of sleeping in; getting out of bed to go into another room when we cant sleep, instead of staying in bed and resting.

The answer: the things you value in life that insomnia – and more particularly your excessive "sleep-safeguarding" - has cost you. The things you valued but don't engage in anymore because you feel you're too tired and lacking in energy to do them.

A values review will highlight for you the reasons you're getting out of bed in the morning, and during the night. In a values review you look at the core areas of your life, their importance to you, and how consistently you live in accord with your values.

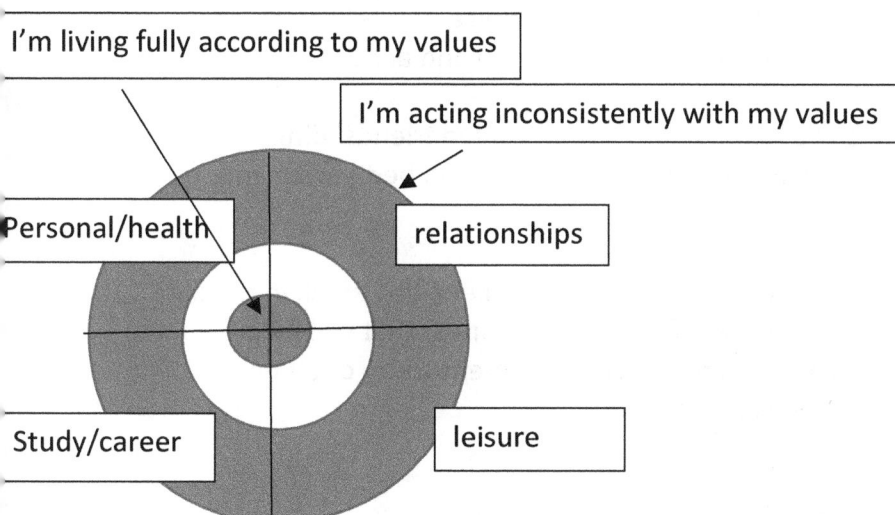

A values bullseye like this (developed by Tobias Lundgren) helps you assess the relative importance of each quadrant of your life and whether you see yourself living fully in line with your values, which gives you a sense of purpose/satisfaction, or not living consistently in line with your values (making for dissatisfaction/ lack of purpose). Think about what you truly value in your life in each area – personal growth/health, study/career, relationships (family/intimate/friendships), and leisure/recreation. You may then start to see a gaping hole between the great importance to you of a few valued areas, and the scarce amount of time and effort in your life that you invest in these compared to chasing sleep.

Let's say your insomnia has driven you to cancel social events in the evening that you never would have cancelled before insomnia hit. You value these friends who've invited you and miss the great times you used to have with them. Your memories of fun shared social events make you resent missing out to "safeguard" your sleep. You realise that being super-careful about your early bedtime has not only cost you opportunities to deepen these relationships, but hasn't improved your sleep quality either.

Immediately you may begin to see how overvaluing sleep, and investing so much time and effort into sleep safety-seeking behaviours (and personal health **is** an important value), is pushing your other values into the background.

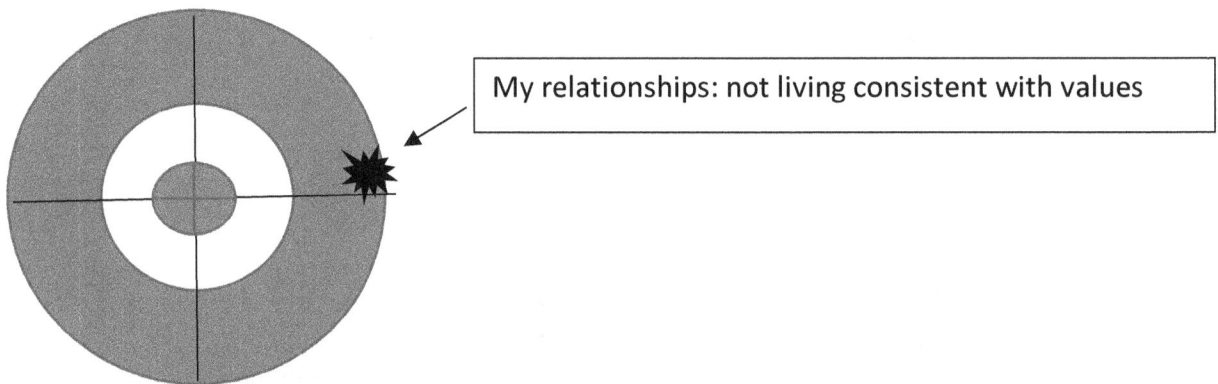

My relationships: not living consistent with values

Now you will inevitably become aware of your other valued areas and the cost of prioritising sleep over all else. And you will find this throws up constant "choice points" day by day where you have to decide what matters more to you to commit to and act on.

So maybe you decide that 6 months is too long to miss out on valued friends' dinners because of sleep efforts that don't work anyway, since you're laying in bed awake and frustrated most nights, and it still takes 1-2 hours to get to sleep.

Sure you have all the HOOKS (thoughts, feelings, memories) that keep you stuck in the old behaviours, but you also have HELPERS (thoughts, feelings, memories) that will help you overturn the old habits, test out your fears, and make a commitment to try out a new direction, because something really valued is at stake.

Your job is to:
1. notice when the choice point hits and how your values are conflicting. You will feel uncomfortable and this is useful in itself.
2. think about how much you value this other area of your life, what you would like it to look like, and how your sleep "safety-seeking" behaviours have distracted you from this.
3. Think about, and record, the "hooks" that hold you back, and the "helpers" that will help motivate you to commit to valued actions.

Your choice point exercise will look like this:

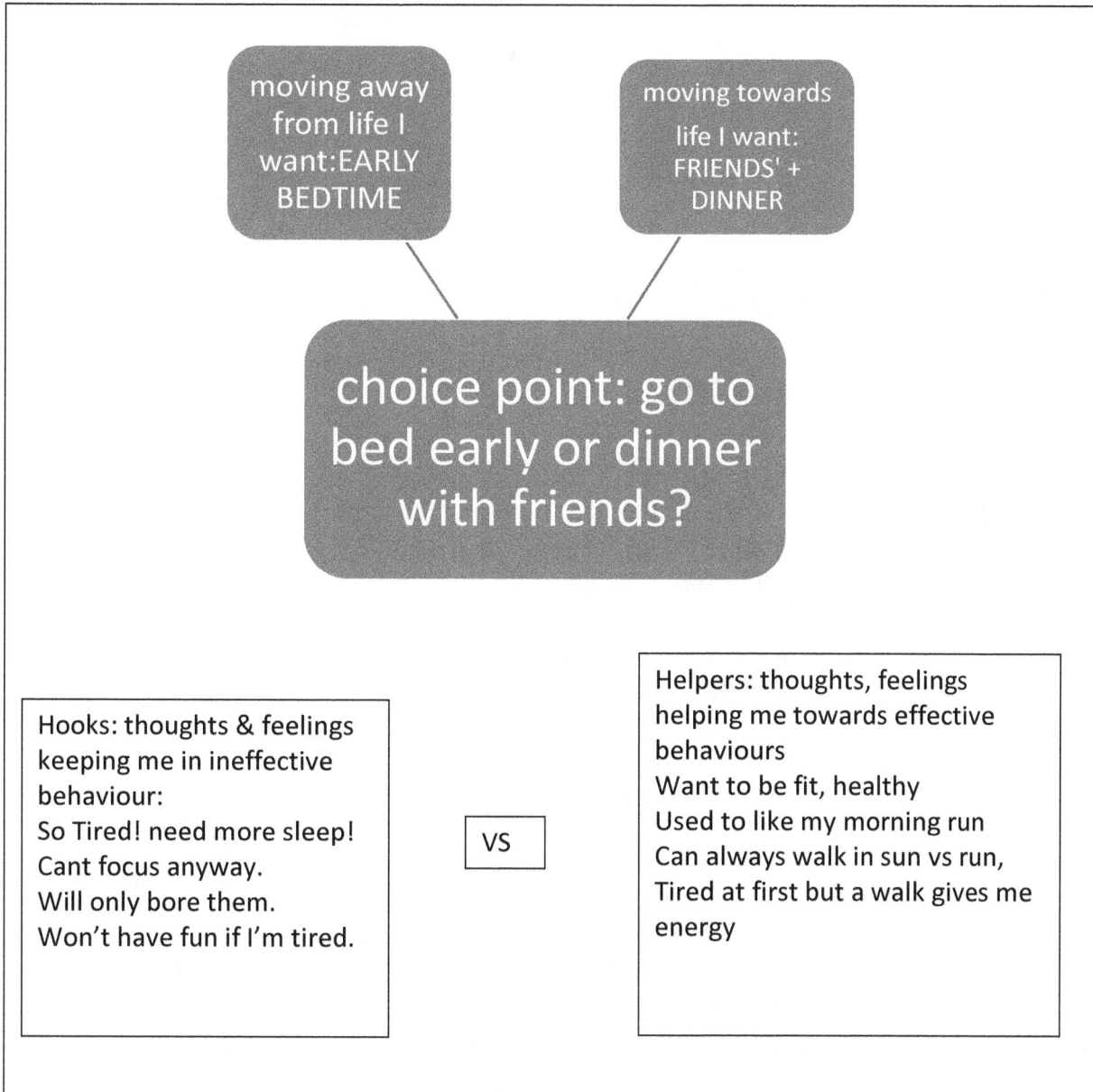

moving away from life I want: EARLY BEDTIME

moving towards life I want: FRIENDS' + DINNER

choice point: go to bed early or dinner with friends?

Hooks: thoughts & feelings keeping me in ineffective behaviour:
So Tired! need more sleep!
Cant focus anyway.
Will only bore them.
Won't have fun if I'm tired.

VS

Helpers: thoughts, feelings helping me towards effective behaviours
Want to be fit, healthy
Used to like my morning run
Can always walk in sun vs run,
Tired at first but a walk gives me energy

```
┌─────────────────┐          ┌─────────────────┐
│  away from      │          │     towards     │
│  life I want:   │          │  life I want: fit &
│  sleep in       │          │  healthy, early │
│                 │          │     rising      │
└────────┬────────┘          └────────┬────────┘
         \                           /
          \                         /
           \                       /
            \                     /
          ┌──────────────────────┐
          │  choice point: get   │
          │  up for a.m. walk    │
          │  or stay in bed?     │
          └──────────────────────┘
```

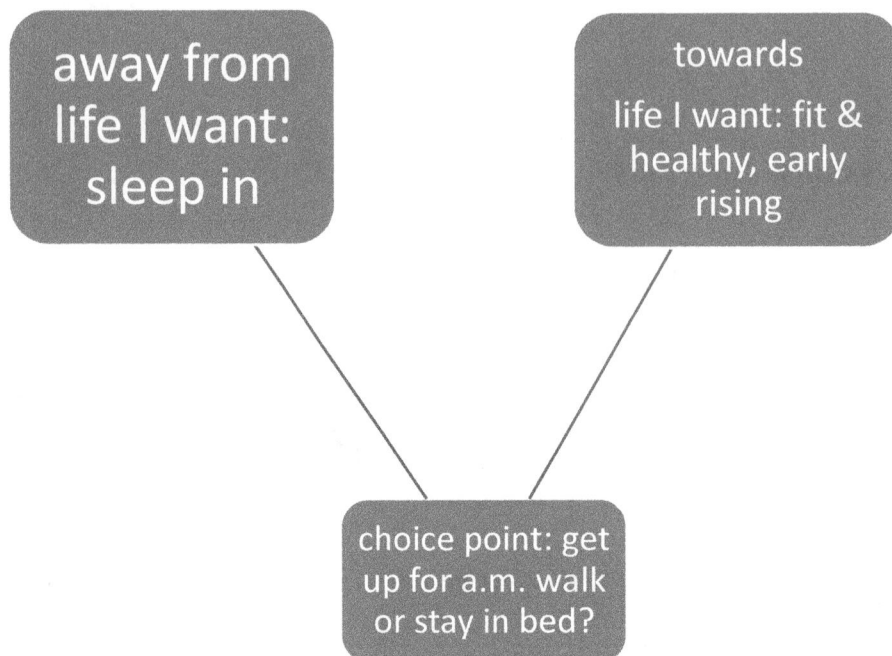

Here's another choice point in insomnia. This one's a bit more difficult because it all involves prioritising your health/personal growth value, but taps into insomnia fears about just *which* actions best reflect the best possible health and self-care.

Here's the reality: The scientific research is saying insufficient sleep is harmful to physical and mental health, not just productivity and work safety (ie, Derk-Jan Dijk, Surrey Sleep Research Centre, David Dinges, University of Pennsylvania; almost everything written about insufficient sleep dangers in the Journals "Sleep", "Hypertension", "Journal of Sleep Research", "JAMA," "Journal of Neurorehabilitation and Neural Repair", etc).
So of course you want to be conscientious and careful for your health. And if this means sleeping in an extra 2 hours until 9am to make up for the 2 hour wakefulness at night, in order to get 8 hours sleep, then that is a good thing, right?

Meanwhile the insomnia CBT research is saying keep to the same waking and rising time daily, and get early morning sunlight, regardless of when you fall asleep or how many hours you sleep, because that will reset your circadian rhythm as well as safeguard your mood.

Because from a chronobiology perspective, if you regularly sleep in that extra 2 hours you may not realise it, but you'll be training your core body temperature to get used to a regular 9am wake-up time. And from a learning perspective you may unexpectedly condition that 2 - 4am wakefulness to your bed if you stay in bed trying to sleep during that time.

This is the hard question: do you prioritise overcoming your insomnia in the longer term even if it means more daytime tiredness and mild sleep deprivation in the short term? Or instead stay in bed to maximise your sleep hours in the short term, even if it means spending 10 hours in bed to get 8 hours sleep (with a conditioned 2-4 am frustrated wakefulness period)? Which one of these looks after your health more?

Because this is an insomnia workbook and the focus is on helping your longterm sleep habits, ideally you'll go with the first option, of getting up early and getting a walk in sunlight.

Let's have a look at the process of weighing up those hooks keeping you in bed, and helpers getting you more sun and earlier waking.

Choice point:	Hooks thoughts & feelings keeping me in ineffective behaviour: stay in bed & sleep in	Helpers thoughts, feelings helping me towards effective behaviours: Get up & walk in sunlight
Do I stay in bed until 9am or get up and walk at 7am?	I'm so tired! My brain says I need to sleep from 7-9am. Those 2 hours sleep are crucial after I've been awake 2 hours. I have to make up for the lost sleep! I need 8 hours sleep, not 6! I feel better after I sleep in 2 more hours – it makes up for the frustration of 2-4am waking.	Want to be fit, healthy. Used to like my morning run & felt good after. If I get up later I won't have time to walk before work. I'm tired but can always walk in sun vs run. Am tired initially but a walk gives me energy for the day. The sun will help my mood. I will probably sleep better tonight since I only got 6 hours last night.

(And just to be even more confusing, the research is also showing that OVERsleeping can affect your risk of mortality. It's not a straightforward linear relationship where more sleep = more health. Once you get past 9 hours of sleep, you increase your risk of poor health and earlier mortality. For example, people with breathing-disordered sleep like Obstructive Sleep Apnoea, may sleep for 10 hours every night but still be at risk because their sleep quality and oxygen saturation levels are so poor).

So have a try working out your own values and how consistently your life aligns with these on the bullseye below. For each area - personal growth/health, study/career, relationships (family/intimate/friendships), and leisure/recreation - ask yourself these questions: "how satisfied am I with this area of my life?"; "what strengths and qualities do I want to develop?"; "do I see a sense of purpose or meaning in this area?"; "is this how I want my life and relationships to look in 5 years?" ; and "what do I want to change about this area of my life?" And for each question, then ask yourself "Has overfocusing on getting my sleep right or conserving energy in the daytime stopped me from developing this area of my life as I want it?" and "Have I been waiting for my sleep to be "right" before I can move forward with my plans in this area?"

MY OWN VALUES AND HOW CLOSELY MY LIFE ALIGNS WITH THESE:

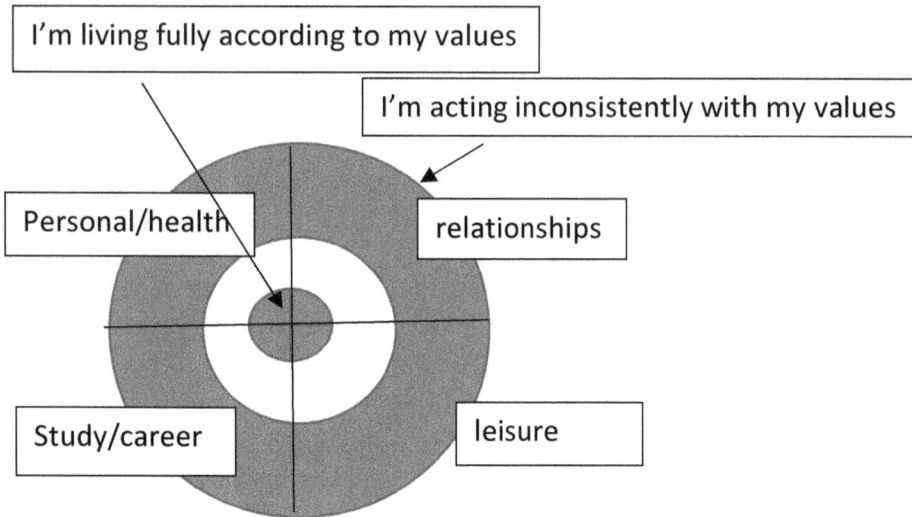

I'm living fully according to my values

I'm acting inconsistently with my values

Personal/health

relationships

Study/career

leisure

Valued areas of my life:	What I value in each area; what each area would look like if I didn't have sleep problems
Personal growth/health:	
Study/career:	
Relationships (family/intimate/friendships):	
Leisure/recreation:	

Now let's have a look at the daily choice points that you can see arising in each area that will make it hard for you to refocus on your valued life and away from insomnia symptoms.

```
┌─────────────────────┐          ┌─────────────────────┐
│  away from life I   │          │    towards the      │
│  want: try to       │          │    life I want:     │
│  sleep/more         │          │                     │
│  time in bed        │          │  Try.................│
└─────────────────────┘          └─────────────────────┘
            \                       /
             \                     /
              \                   /
           ┌─────────────────────┐
           │  choice point: Do   │
           │  ..............? or try │
           │  to sleep More?     │
           └─────────────────────┘
```

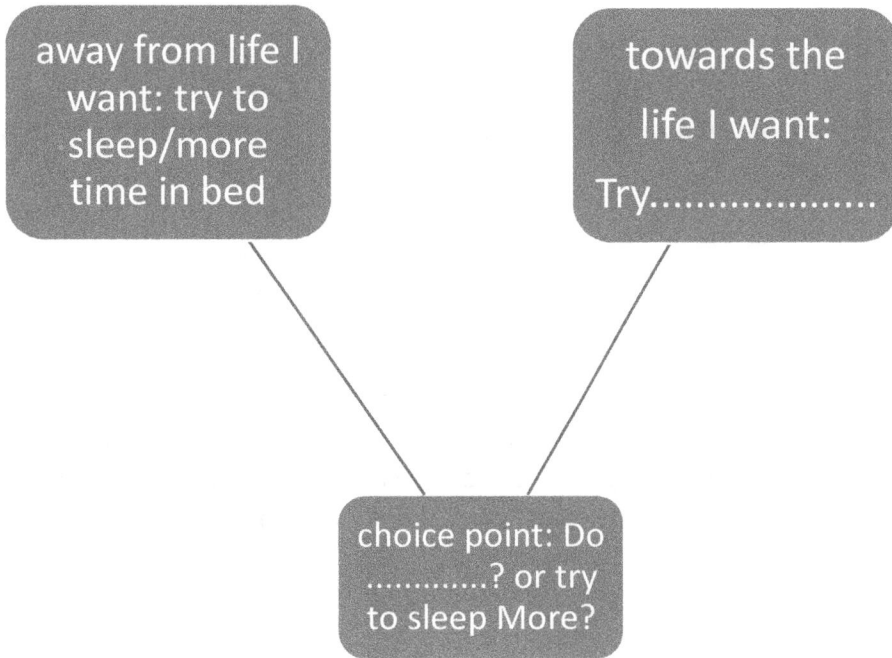

Let's have a look at the process of weighing up those hooks keeping you in bed, and helpers getting you more sun and earlier waking.

Choice point:	Hooks thoughts & feelings keeping me in ineffective behaviour: stay in bed & sleep in	Helpers thoughts, feelings helping me towards effective behaviours: Try……………………………..
Do I stay in bed, try to get more sleep? or try…………… Instead?	I'm so tired! If I feel tired I must need sleep! I have to make up for the lost sleep! I need 8 hours sleep, not …! I feel better after I sleep in.. Every hour counts!	

NB: this exercise is for people with insomnia, (ie with worry, hypervigilance and sleep-seeking behaviours, to try out). This exercise is expressly not intended for anyone with a history of mania or hypomania who may UNDERvalue sleep and instead value/prioritise excitement-tinged activities over sleep.

In summary:

The aim of this chapter is to review our values in order to help us *want* to try the sleep behaviour changes. Not to feel pressured to *have* to change. *Have-to* goals feel like a punishment and imposition, prompted by fear ("..but I really feel the best solution is to sleep until 10am because the researchers say 7 hours sleep is the absolute minimum, and morning's when I can finally get some sleep! Why would I want early morning sunlight?").

Want-to goals reflect our true values (our "whys"). We work on these difficult sleep changes because of the inherent importance to us of longterm sleep habits, not quick fixes. We freely choose these goals because we see good sleep as an important quality that helps us feel good and enjoy life. "Sure, it's hard gradually reducing these sleep medications and putting up with the dream sleep rebound, but I want to get back to sleeping without medications because I actually felt better and healthier before them."

The major difference between these want-to vs have-to reasons is that although *have-to* motivations will allow us to make positive changes for a while, eventually that determination is going to break down.

Want-to motivation is actually associated with lower automatic attraction toward the cues that will hook you back into old habits. It instead pulls you towards actions that will help you achieve your goals. *Have-to* motivation actually increases temptation because it makes you feel constricted or deprived. So doing a behaviour change for *have-to* reasons will likely undermine your self-control and make you more vulnerable to keep doing unhelpful actions. Your attention will always be focused on feeling imposed on by stupid arbitrary rules, and not feeling agency over your own life. Imagine the difference between "It's hard to get up early and walk in the morning but it sets me up for the day and I get more done" compared to "Why do I have to get up at the same time every morning for sunlight? I'm only doing it because it's my homework; I'm definitely going to sleep in until midday on the weekend, I deserve a break".

Knowing your "whys" and living in accordance with your values, makes all the difference to your sleep.

PART 3: UNLEARNING SLEEP MEDICATION DEPENDENCE:

Charles Morin in 2004 found that nine out of 10 subjects who combined a gradual reduction in their medication with InsomniaCBT were drug-free after seven weeks. Only half of those who tried to stop using the pills just by reducing dose alone were as successful. Doing InsomniaCBT before and during gradual medication tapering significantly improves success rate and likelihood of maintaining treatment gains, because core beliefs and expectations about sleep are changed longterm.

CHAPTER 12: COLLABORATING WITH YOUR PRESCRIBER:

BENZODIAZEPINES BENEFITS & RISKS

In the 20-year (1992-2011) period, 174 080 904 scripts were dispensed in Australia, with temazepam the most dispensed benzodiazepine (35% of scripts), followed by diazepam (23%). Since 1998, there has been a modest but steady increase in per-script DDD, or World Health Organization-defined daily doses.

BENZODIAZEPINE BENEFITS

Benzodiazepines are used for insomnia, anxiety, reducing muscle tension and other situations where there is a need to calm or sedate the central nervous system.

The need for benzodiazepines -short term- in *acute* psychiatric emergencies, anaesthesia, intensive care, palliative care at the end of life, and in the treatment of seizures and alcohol withdrawal is accepted as objectively beneficial. But it is their long-term use for anxiety and insomnia that is increasingly questioned. As Malcolm Lader of the Addiction Research Centre at King's College states: "The risk-benefit ratio of the benzodiazepines remains positive in most patients in the short term (2-4 weeks) but is unestablished beyond that time, due mainly to the difficulty in preventing short-term use from extending indefinitely with the risk of dependence." (Lader, 2011, Addictions).

BENZODIAZEPINES RISKS

Although safe in the short term some risks have been noted with the sleep medications (both benzodiazepines and BZRAs eg Stilnox and Imovane). Tolerance building & associated disorganised, ad hoc self-medicating behaviours; unwitting extra doses leading to accidental overdose because of therapeutic amnesia; next-day sedation & motor vehicle accidents (on the basis of this the US Food & Drug Administration issued a guideline to manufacturers to halve the recommended starting dose of the BZRA Zopiclone in 2013).

Sleeping pills contribute to mortality risk through fatal motor vehicle accidents, as noted by Neuroscientist Matthew Walker in "Why We Sleep". He cites the pills' non-restorative sleep and/or groggy hangover creating next day drowsiness while driving. The Australian Sleep Health Foundation also linked motor vehicle accidents to sleep problems and next day sedation.

The Victorian Coroners Court produced a 2015 report, citing benzodiazepine involvement in 43% of overdose fatalities (Xanax and Valium have since been moved to Schedule 8 restricted drugs). Benzodiazepines are the most common drug found in drug deaths in Australia, and most drug deaths in Australia are accidental (Australian Bureau of Statistics, 2016).

Benzodiazepines can cause confusion, cognitive impairment, balance problems and falls, generating significant socioeconomic costs. The risks increase with advancing age, and use is more common in older adults. Australia's population is ageing, living longer with more insomnia and associated anxiety just as physical frailty, mobility and balance problems increase as problems. Thus benzodiazepine effects are an increasing concern.

ACCIDENTAL OVERDOSE RISK

In 2016 the Australian Bureau of Statistics released data showing benzodiazepines were the most common substance present in drug related deaths in that year, being identified in 663 (36.7%) deaths. Benzodiazepines were the most common drug in both unintentional and suicidal drug deaths in 2016. The researchers found that the vast majority (approximately 66%) of drug deaths were accidental rather than intentional.

Benzodiazepines were the most common substance in drug deaths for women from age 20 to their mid-60s, and were the most common substance present in deaths of men in the 35-39 age group.

In over 96% of drug deaths where benzodiazepines were present in 2016, they were taken in conjunction with other drugs including alcohol. The Bureau cautioned that benzodiazepines can be dangerous when taken with other substances as they affect the central nervous system and risk causing respiratory depression. And barring 1999 (when prescription opioids were the single most identified substances in drug induced deaths) the consistent most common single substance identified on drug fatality toxicology reports has been benzodiazepines.

Meanwhile, over in the United States, the National Institute on Drug Abuse reported that, compared with 1,135 total Benzodiazepine overdose deaths in 1999, there were 10,684 overdose deaths involving benzodiazepines in the United States in 2016.

The Morbidity and Mortality Weekly Report of January 11, 2019, showed an 830% rise in the number of overdose deaths involving benzodiazepines among women aged 30 to 64 from 1999 to 2017 (ie, from 0.54 per 100,000 in 1999 to 5.02 per 100,000 in 2017).

The researchers cited benzodiazepines' sedating effect, particularly dangerous when used with other drugs (like opiates and alcohol) that slow breathing. In combination, the substances can lead "people to fall asleep and essentially never wake up again", according to Stanford University School of Medicine addiction psychiatrist Anna Lembke.

Unfortunately the attribution change that tends to happen with continued sleep prescription medication use increases the risks. Along with the tolerance effects of anxiety symptom and insomnia return, and the therapeutic amnesia that we don't seem able to lessen over time, the attributions of an external agent "looking after" our sleep (when we believe our brains can't) leads us into sometimes desperate ad hoc self-medicating actions. Intermittent reinforcement or sleep reward on medications, accentuated as tolerance develops, promotes escalation of frantic sleep safety-seeking behaviours with increasing learned helplessness, anxiety and uncertainty about sleep outcomes.

DEPENDENCE

When insomnia patients use sleeping pills for a few weeks, even at low dose this tends to cause physiological dependence (both tolerance and withdrawal). Tolerance refers to the effect of the drug wearing off over time, with a higher dose needed for the same effect. Upon stopping the pills users often have severe withdrawal symptoms – the very insomnia they were trying to avoid, but also irritability, muscle tension, headache, panic attacks, tremor, sweating, poor concentration, nausea, rapid heart rate. Stopping too suddenly after longterm use can cause seizures, so it's very important to work with a medical professional to reduce gradually. Understandably, longterm use is not recommended because the side effects and withdrawal effects are well-known in the medical community.

WHAT THE MEDICAL BODIES SAY

In 2016 The American College of Physicians strongly recommended, after evaluating the efficacy and safety of cognitive behaviour therapy (CBT-I) against standard sleep medications, that CBT-I must be the first line treatment for all chronic insomnia cases, not sleeping pills. (Published in Annals of Internal Medicine).

In Australia the RACGP (Royal Australian College of General Practitioners) also publishes benzodiazepine prescribing guidelines stating CBT must be the first line treatment for chronic insomnia, not sleeping pills.

CBT works to teach people good sleep habits, and manage expectations, to prevent unhelpful coping behaviours & distrust around sleep and the bed environment. Hypnotic (sleep-inducing) prescription medications are still the cheapest, most prevalent "go to" insomnia treatment, but tend to reinforce an external locus of control, and external attribution of sleep success. This tends to reduce rather than increase insomnia sufferers' sense of agency or self-mastery. These medications also have potential to affect sleep architecture, suppressing dream sleep necessary for memory consolidation, & reducing slow-wave (deep) sleep, necessary for tissue and cell repair, human growth hormone production, and immune health.

Apart from the risk of physiological dependence the main reason sleeping pills can inadvertently become insomnia-prolonging is psychological. Each of us has a "locus of control" - a subjective perception that our actions are motivated either via our internal resources or by externally imposed forces. People who take prescription sleep medication regularly tend to have an external locus of control around sleep. They tend to attribute their sleep success to the pill rather than their own efforts. As a result they also tend to believe they are themselves unable to sleep on their own. This interacts with physical withdrawal so that a night without sleeping pills leads to expectations of poor sleep, leads to tension and frustration in bed. This becomes a self-fulfilling prophecy where the agitation and helplessness feelings confirm the need to get back on the medication.

This can even lead to a circular logic of one insomnia patient who stated "I've been on medications so long now my sleep must be broken, so now I'll need to stay on medications for the rest of my life". He genuinely believed the medications had "taken over" sleep regulation and his brain would now be unable to achieve sleep on its own.

In reality the medication is not "taking over" sleep; users who want sleep still need to enter a "collaborative" process with the medication (as Glovinsky & Spielman describe it) and play a role in calming their own nervous system and racing mind in order for the sedation to invite the sleep process. The user is the one who decides to let sleep happen, allowing the medication to sedate, or resisting its effects.

Once attributions are changed we can see almost obsessive nightly decision-making and experimenting before bedtime with sleep medications (for example, the actor Heath Ledger's lethal mix of CNS-depressant hypnotics, antihistamines, analgesics, and opiates). This "cements" a trap: higher expectations ("it should be working!"), create more attention to sleep, and more anxiety about sleep, not less. This is how sleep medications become part of the circular hypervigilance loop of insomnia. People with insomnia value sleep more, think more about it, and expect more from sleep. Requiring sleep to make them feel refreshed, energetic, focused and happy is too much pressure for the brain to bear.

The cognitive and attentional bias toward catastrophe is also apparent when REM sleep rebound occurs upon withdrawing from benzodiazepines after an extended period of daily use. This is another reason to very slowly and gradually taper benzodiazepine use. Because benzodiazepines may have suppressed REM or dream sleep over an extended period, users are alarmed to experience more vivid and startling dreams over the period that REM sleep is recovered by the brain. If the insomnia sufferer could expect this REM rebound to be likely it could reduce fear, and reduce the urge to go straight back on the medication to prevent the dream content.

It would be even better to reframe this rebound dream sleep as healthy, with the brain reasserting its need for dream sleep (for memory consolidation and emotion regulation) and taking the upper hand in regulating sleep as it evolved to do. Thinking of the REM rebound in this way would go a long way to calming fears about what the dreams represent.

Expectations: it should work!

I need refreshing sleep.

I can't do it alone.

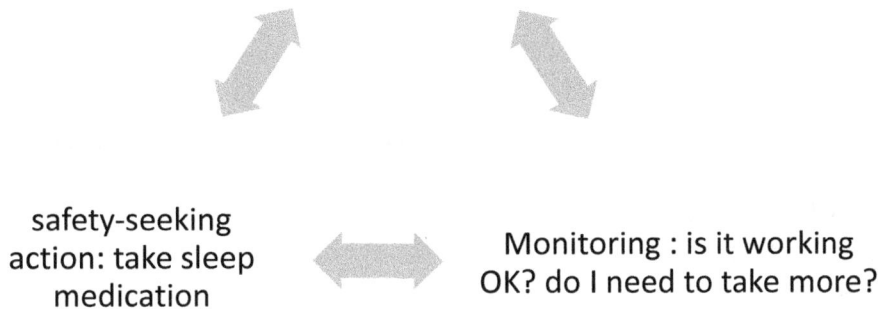

safety-seeking
action: take sleep
medication

Monitoring : is it working
OK? do I need to take more?

In this vicious hypervigilance loop, where to start working?

Answer: While you start discussions with your doctor to gradually reduce sleep medications, we will start work on your sleep expectations, because expectations about sleep will decide whether or not you overestimate threat – about sleep loss and next day functioning. And whether you are wide awake at 2am or tired and wired at 11am, we can start looking at how you attribute sleep success and failure.

Reflect for a moment: What are my own attributions about medications and sleep? What do I attribute the good sleeps to – the sleep medication or my own sleep self-regulation processes? What do I attribute the poor sleeps to – the sleep medication or my own sleep self-regulation processes?

My Expectations:
(shoulds):

Monitoring : (attention):

sleep safety-
seeking action:
take medication

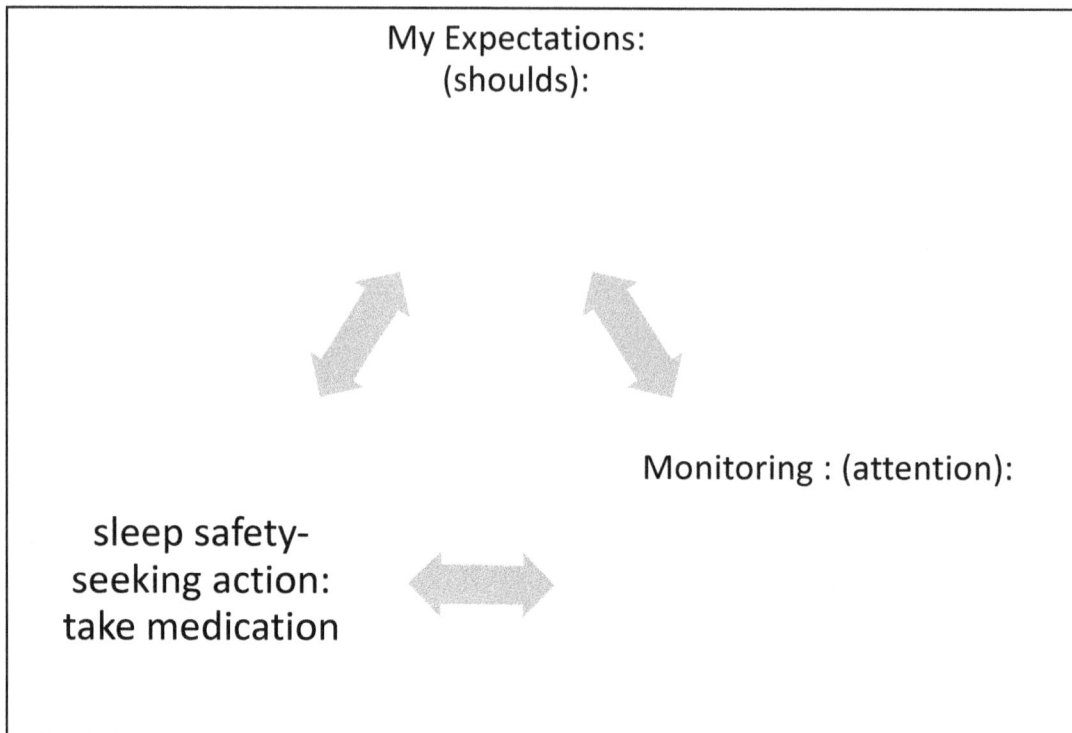

BENZODIAZEPINE REDUCTION SCHEDULES

COLLABORATING WITH YOUR DOCTOR TO REDUCE SLEEP MEDICATION DEPENDENCE

Even benzodiazepine use at the prescribed dose for as little as 3 to 6 weeks has been associated with developing physical dependence. Between 15–44% of chronic benzodiazepine users may experience drawn-out moderate to severe withdrawal symptoms upon stopping, including break-through anxiety and depression symptoms. Not everyone finds the process overwhelming. In longer term use of more than 6 months, approximately 40% of benzodiazepine users will have a moderate to severe withdrawal, and perhaps 60% will have a quite mild withdrawal syndrome, if stopping rapidly.

Generally however, it's important not to abruptly stop taking benzodiazepines, or even taper too quickly, because of withdrawal symptoms that could create distress (anxiety symptoms, sleeplessness, perceptual distortions) and if more severe, potential central nervous system damage. Severe benzodiazepine withdrawal symptoms can resemble acute alcohol withdrawal, with DT's (delirium tremens), seizures, psychosis, and hallucinations.

Gradual tapering of doses, even in milligram reductions for weeks at a time with some benzodiazepine types, are the best way to reduce the discomfort of withdrawal. The central nervous system will take time to adjust after benzodiazepine withdrawal, taking from 6-18 months to achieve full recovery. The online Ashton Manual shows tables that provide multiple detailed examples of moving from highly addictive short-acting benzodiazepines to safer longer-acting benzodiazepines over many months, reducing by milligrams at a time. This can regularly take over 50-70 weeks in many (20-35) stages of 1-2 weeks each. (There will be more detail at the end of this chapter). It is a good idea to maximise chances of success by getting ongoing supportive counselling, or even better, 1:1 cognitive behaviour therapy (CBT), to cope during planned withdrawal.

Please start by visiting the website www.benzo.org.uk/index.htm and carefully reading the slow withdrawal schedules. Then print out a guideline that incorporates the benzodiazepine medication you are taken and take that to your doctor as a starting point. If you are on multiple medications it will be important to make a list of these and any herbal or over-the-counter preparations your doctor may not know about.

It will be essential to work on this process with your prescribing doctor in case you are not coping with the withdrawal rate and need to supplement the dose temporarily to cope with symptoms. It won't be sufficient to use this workbook for the whole process. After doing the insomnia CBT program you will have a psychological starting point for working with your prescriber to start gradual dose reduction. There is no book that will be able to substitute for the individualized advice of your prescribing doctor who can modify the tapering schedule to work with your own needs and incorporate other information (such as the other substances or medications you are taking which might affect the withdrawal process).

SUBSTITUTING BENZODIAZEPINES BEFORE TAPERING

For safety and a less distressing reduction program your doctor may want to substitute a short-acting benzodiazepine like lorazepam for a long-acting benzodiazepine like diazepam(valium). The long-acting pills have a slow onset and long half-life, compared to the short-acting fast-onset pills, which are harder to taper off because they are very reinforcing to your brain's reward pathways. (tolerance builds faster because the user experiences faster withdrawal and immediately seeks more and more of the substance to get the same effect).

Remember the slow tapering schedule lets your body and mind successfully adjust to each new reduction level and gradually return to normal functioning.

In the meantime you will have been using CBT-I to learning thinking and habit changes that will help you to genuinely overcome sleep fears longterm, and attribute good sleep to your own mastery, not an external medication.

REASONS TO COME OFF BENZODIAZEPINE SLEEP MEDICATIONS
In summary, apart from the reassuring evidence about your brain's natural sleep regulation processes from the CBT-I program, there are a number of good reasons to wean off medications while treating insomnia:

1. Using the pills longterm will probably make you feel worse and more generally anxious as tolerance builds and your brai's neural pathways adapt to the medication.
2. People often feel helpless, frustrated, depressed and low in self-esteem if they perceive that they are trapped on medications and not learning skills or mastery.
3. Your sleep quality will likely be affected over time if you use these medications longterm, due to REM sleep suppression and effects on Slow-Wave (deep) sleep.
4. With tolerance building over time the pills are unlikely to be an effective solution in the long term– you'll be getting central nervous system sedation but not enough actual sleep.
5. Dependence shows up as tolerance effects and "break-through" withdrawal effects (physical and mental) despite continued use.
6. Benzodiazepine side effects create real risk as you get older: balance problems, confusion, memory loss, falls risk.
7. There is evidence emerging of increased dementia risk in longterm users.
8. On the plus side, not everyone experiences a difficult withdrawal; with careful medication substitution, withdrawal effects can be kept to a bearable level, and the feelings of mastery and achievement for weaning off dependency are significant.

Internal debate about tapering off my prescription sleep medication:	
Pros of staying on same medication level	Cons of staying on same medication level
Pros of tapering off sleep medication	Cons of tapering off sleep medication

What are the reasons I will discuss with my doctor for reducing or tapering off sleep medication?

....
....
....
....

What kind of exit planning for these medications do I want to discuss with my doctor?

....

....

....

....

DO I REDUCE OUTSIDE OR INSIDE HOSPITAL?

Tapering benzodiazepines is also known as "weaning" off these medications. If you are doing this outside of hospital your doctor may recommend reducing by 10% every 1-2 weeks. However this outpatient approach won't work if you have an established dependence where you frequently respond to tolerance by kneejerk self-medicating under stress. Especially if you have existing memory problems. It isn't uncommon for doctors to collaborate on an 8-10 week program on reducing sleep medications only to find the patient has taken all the medications by day 4 of the program. These patients will need an inpatient detox.

Discussions with my prescribing doctor about outpatient or inpatient (clinic) detox:	
Pros of detoxing in clinic	Cons of detoxing in clinic
Pros of detoxing as an outpatient long term	Cons of detoxing as an outpatient long term

INPATIENT TAPERING SCHEDULE

An inpatient detox in an addictions ward can reduce benzodiazepine doses much faster while managing the withdrawal effects safely. Charles Duhigg also writes, in terms of breaking a habit: outside of your normal environment, the cues driving habits change, so you have a "clean slate" and fresh chance to break out of a habit and change the cue-habit-reward loop. Potentially an inpatient detox can be this "clean slate" away from home environment cues driving old habitual actions.

Your doctor may well err on the side of caution and book you in for this medically supervised withdrawal if you have been benzodiazepine-dependent for a long time or there are indications that you may have an increased seizure risk.

Here are some medication reduction fundamentals to discuss with your doctor:

You and your doctor will collaborate on how to go about this, and a reduction procedure may look something like:

1. First stabilising on a normal daily dose and ensure that the dose is taken regularly throughout the day (so no ad hoc changes based on feeling states or anxiety levels);
2. Your doctor will advise on whether and how to change a more addictive short-acting benzodiazepine to a less addictive long-acting one like diazepam
3. Reducing by a small amount of one dose (your doctor may suggest 10% of the overall dose)
4. Then stabilising on the reduced amount for at least two weeks, again trying to stabilise with no variations or ad hoc changes based on feeling states (unless stressful life events;
5. Reviewing with your doctor every 2 weeks or more frequently to discuss withdrawal symptom levels and coping ability,
6. Then reducing again after review by an amount that is calibrated to maximise coping ability and symptom manageability;
7. Regular reviews fortnightly or weekly with your doctor to monitor progress and coping, taking "rests" during the reduction process if the physical and psychological symptoms are too severe, or during stressful life events that overwhelm your coping ability.
8. Recording self-mastery ratings and attribution thoughts on your thought record to generate internal motivation to keep going.

The Ashton Manual online (at Benzo.org – see https://www.benzo.org.uk/manual/) has many sample schedules of safe, gradual benzodiazepine reduction schedules. Print out an example that reflects your medication use to take to your doctor and start the discussion.

The schedule overleaf is just an example of a tapering schedule. **Under no circumstances should you see this as a prescription for you to follow: you and your doctor will necessarily devise your own individualised schedule based on many factors that relate only to you and your health and circumstances.** This is simply an example to provide a realistic picture of how long the process often takes, in order to avoid panic and increase success likelihood.

Schedule 2. Simple withdrawal from diazepam (Valium) 40mg daily
(follow this schedule to complete Schedule 1)

	Morning	Night	Total Daily Dosage
Starting dosage	diazepam 20mg	diazepam 20mg	40mg
Stage 1 (1-2 weeks)	diazepam 18mg	diazepam 20mg	38mg
Stage 2 (1-2 weeks)	diazepam 18mg	diazepam 18mg	36mg
Stage 3 (1-2 weeks)	diazepam 16mg	diazepam 18mg	34mg
Stage 4 (1-2 weeks)	diazepam 16mg	diazepam 16mg	32mg
Stage 5 (1-2 weeks)	diazepam 14mg	diazepam 16mg	30mg
Stage 6 (1-2 weeks)	diazepam 14mg	diazepam 14mg	28mg
Stage 7 (1-2 weeks)	diazepam 12mg	diazepam 14mg	26mg
Stage 8 (1-2 weeks)	diazepam 12mg	diazepam 12mg	24mg
Stage 9 (1-2 weeks)	diazepam 10mg	diazepam 12mg	22mg
Stage 10 (1-2 weeks)	diazepam 10mg	diazepam 10mg	20mg
Stage 11 (1-2 weeks)	diazepam 8mg	diazepam 10mg	18mg
Stage 12 (1-2 weeks)	diazepam 8mg	diazepam 8mg	16mg
Stage 13 (1-2 weeks)	diazepam 6mg	diazepam 8mg	14mg
Stage 14 (1-2 weeks)	diazepam 5mg	diazepam 8mg	13mg
Stage 15 (1-2 weeks)	diazepam 4mg	diazepam 8mg	12mg
Stage 16 (1-2 weeks)	diazepam 3mg	diazepam 8mg	11mg
Stage 17 (1-2 weeks)	diazepam 2mg	diazepam 8mg	10mg
Stage 18 (1-2 weeks)	diazepam 1mg	diazepam 8mg	9mg
Stage 19 (1-2 weeks)	--	diazepam 8mg	8mg
Stage 20 (1-2 weeks)	--	diazepam 7mg	7mg
Stage 21 (1-2 weeks)	--	diazepam 6mg	6mg
Stage 22 (1-2 weeks)	--	diazepam 5mg	5mg
Stage 23 (1-2 weeks)	--	diazepam 4mg	4mg
Stage 24 (1-2 weeks)	--	diazepam 3mg	3mg
Stage 25 (1-2 weeks)	--	diazepam 2mg	2mg
Stage 26 (1-2 weeks)	--	diazepam 1mg	1mg

Each Schedule in the online Manual has notes attached to help you anticipate difficulties and discuss these with your doctor. Again, the above schedule and dosing is hypothetical and merely illustrates what a schedule may look like.

The important part is planning out your own best-fit schedule in collaboration with your doctor:

My tapering schedule:		Morning	Night	Total daily dose
Starting dose	Weeks on	.........(eg 10mg)	.........(eg 10mg)	20mg
Stage 1	1-2 weeks			
Stage 2				
Stage 3				
Stage 4				
Stage 5				
Stage 6				
Stage 7				
Stage 8				
Stage 9				
Stage 10				
Stage 11				
Stage 12				
Stage 13				
Stage 14				
Stage 15				
Stage 16				
Stage 17				
Stage 18				
Stage 19				
Stage 20				
Stage 21				
Stage 22				
Stage 23				
Stage 24	2 weeks			
Stage 25	2 weeks			
Stage 26	2 weeks			
Stage Etc.				
Contract Signed:	Me:		Dr:	
	Date: / /		Date: / /	

FURTHER ADVICE & SUPPORT ONLINE:

Benzodiazepine Dependence, Toxicity and Abuse: American Psychiatric Association

The Ashton Manual Supplement: How Benzodiazepines Work and How to Withdraw (2002)

The Ashton Manual - Benzo.org: https://www.benzo.org.uk/manual/

FURTHER READING:

Buysse, D, SLEEP, 2014; 37 (1):9-17

Daniel J. Buysse, M.D., Anne Germain, Ph.D., Martica Hall, Ph.D., Timothy H. Monk, D.Sc., Ph.D., and Eric A. Nofzinger, M.D. "A Neurobiological Model of Insomnia" January 2012

Chambers, M. J. and Keller, B. Alert insomniacs: are they really sleep deprived? Clin. Psychol. Rev., 1993, 13: 649–666

Colin Espie "Overcoming Insomnia and Sleep Problems". Robinson: UK 2010.

Colin A. Espie Clinical Psychologist. "ABC of sleep disorders. Practical management of insomnia: behavioural and cognitive techniques." February, 1993

Duhigg, C "The Power of Habit" 2012. Random House Books.

Karen Falloon, PhD Candidate, Bruce Arroll, Professor and Head of Department, C Raina Elley, Associate Professor, Antonio Fernando III, Senior Lecturer2. "ABC of sleep disorders. Practical management of insomnia: behavioural and cognitive techniques." April 2011

Freedman NS, Kotzer N, Schwab RJ. Patient perception of sleep quality and etiology of sleep disruption in the intensive care unit. Am J Respir Crit Care Med. 1999 Apr;159(4 Pt 1):1155-62.

Freedman NS, Gazendam J, Levan L, Pack AI, Schwab RJ. Abnormal sleep/wake cycles and the effect of environmental noise on sleep disruption in the intensive care unit. Am J Respir Crit Care Med. 2001 Feb;163(2):451-7.

Harvey, A., Murray, Chandler, Soehner, 2010, Sleep Disturbance as a mechanism in causing symptoms and disability in multiple psychiatric problems.

Jastreboff, P. & Hazell, J. (2008) Tinnitus Retraining Therapy: Implementing the Neurophysiological Model. Cambridge University Press.
Leon C. Lack & Helen R. Wright. Clinical Management of Delayed Sleep Phase Disorder. Behavioural Sleep Medicine. Pages 57-76: 05 Dec 2007

Leon C. Lack, Helen R. Wright, PhD, Richard R. Bootzin, Delayed Sleep-Phase Disorder, Sleep Medicine Clinics, June 2009,Volume 4, Issue 2, Pages 229–239

Mejo SL. Anterograde amnesia linked to benzodiazepines. Nurse Pract. 1992 Oct;17(10):44, 49-50.

Christopher B. Miller PhD. Institute of Neuroscience and Psychology, Woolcock Institute of Medical Research. "Sleep restriction therapy: experimental studies" June 2014

Morin, Charles. Espie, C. Insomnia: a Clinical Guide to Assessment and Treatment, Kluwer Aademic/Plenum Press: New York, 2003.

Qaseem A, Kansagara D, Forciea MA, Cooke M, Denberg TD; Clinical Guidelines Committee of the American College of Physicians. Management of Chronic Insomnia Disorder in Adults: A Clinical Practice Guideline From the American College of Physicians. Ann Intern Med. 2016 Jul 19;165(2):125-33. doi: 10.7326/M15-2175. Epub 2016 May 3.

Ree, M. and Harvey, A (2004). Insomnia. In Bennett-Levy, J. Butler, G., Fennell, M. Hackmann, A. Mueller, M. & Westbrook, D. Oxford Guide to Behavioural Expriments in cognitive Therapy. Oxford University Press.

Riemann, Baglioni , Bassetti , Bjorvatn, Dolenc Groselj , Ellis, Espie C, Garcia-Borreguero D, Gjerstad M, Gonçalves M, Hertenstein E, Jansson-Fröjmark M, Jennum PJ, Leger D, Nissen C, Parrino L, Paunio T, Pevernagie D, Verbraecken J, Weeß HG, Wichniak A, Zavalko I, Arnardottir E, Deleanu O, Strazisar B, Zoetmulder M, Spiegelhalder . European guideline for the diagnosis and treatment of insomnia. J Sleep Res. 2017 Dec;26(6):675-700. doi: 10.1111/jsr.12594. Epub 2017 Sep 5.

Julia M. Selfridge, Tetsuya Gotoh, Samuel Schiffhauer, JingJing Liu, Philip E. Stauffer, Andrew Li, Daniel G. S. Capelluto, and Carla V. Finkielstein . "Chronotherapy: Intuitive, Sound, Founded...But Not Broadly Applied". Drugs. 2016; 76(16): 1507–1521.

Tyler, R.S. and Baker L.J. (1983) Difficulties experienced by tinnitus sufferers. J.Speech Hear. Disord., 48,150-154.

Valenzuela, C.F. (1997) Alcohol and Neurotransmitter Interactions. Alcohol Health & Research World. Vol 21, No.2, 144-148.

Vinkers, CH and Olivier, B. Mechanisms Underlying Tolerance after Long-Term Benzodiazepine Use: A Future for Subtype-Selective GABAA Receptor Modulators? Advances in Pharmacological Science.Published online 2012 Mar 29.

Sean David Hood, Amanda Norman, Dana Adelle Hince, Jan Krzysztof Melichar,Gary Kenneth Hulse. Benzodiazepine dependence and its treatment with low dose flumazenil. Br J Clin Pharmacol. 2014 Feb; 77(2): 285–294.

ORGANISATIONS OFFERING FURTHER INFORMATION & SUPPORT:
www.adt-healthcare.com/blog/post/guide-to-safely-withdrawing-benzodiazepines
http://www.reconnexion.org.au/research
Benzo-Wise: A recovery Companion: V. Baylissa Frederick

CBT SLEEP APPS & WEBSITES:
UK: Sleepio.com /USA: Shut-*i* / NHS: Sleepstation/ Australia: Sleepfit

www.ingramcontent.com/pod-product-compliance
Lightning Source LLC
Chambersburg PA
CBHW08085803426
42334CB00022B/2622